As a practicing neurointerventional surgeon in San Diego and colleague of Dr. Levy, I was utterly captivated by the compelling and personal nature of these clinical vignettes. It takes both courage and personal fortitude to openly discuss one's spiritual beliefs in this high-stakes and often cynical field. I can personally attest to the compassion, humility, and prowess I have witnessed in David's practice. While he and I come from different religious backgrounds, I found the humanistic qualities of his work to be broadly applicable and inspirational to caregivers from all walks of life.

JORDAN ZIEGLER, MD
San Diego

Dr. Levy is a well-trained, experienced, and professionally superb brain surgeon. In bringing God into the equation, he has broken through a near-taboo, and he has done so for the good of patient and family. To do such good is the essence of our calling; for another physician, an agnostic, to recognize his accomplishment must be the highest compliment. You will enjoy this book and the gift of insight it gives you.

CHARLES KERBER, MD
Professor of Radiology and Neurosurgery
UCSD Medical Center
San Diego

Neurosurgery can be extraordinarily stressful, both for patients and physicians, but in the book *Gray Matter* neurosurgeon David Levy shows us how spirituality can help defuse some of the tension, while providing readers with a very interesting educational perspective on the brain and its potential. I am delighted to have one of my colleagues stand up boldly for faith and intellect.

BENJAMIN S. CARSON SR., MD

The Benjamin S. Carson Sr., MD, and Dr. Evelyn Spiro, RN,
Professor of Pediatric Neurosurgery
Director of Pediatric Neurosurgery
Professor of Neurological Surgery, Oncology, Plastic Surgery, and Pediatrics
Johns Hopkins Medical Institutions
Author of Gifted Hands

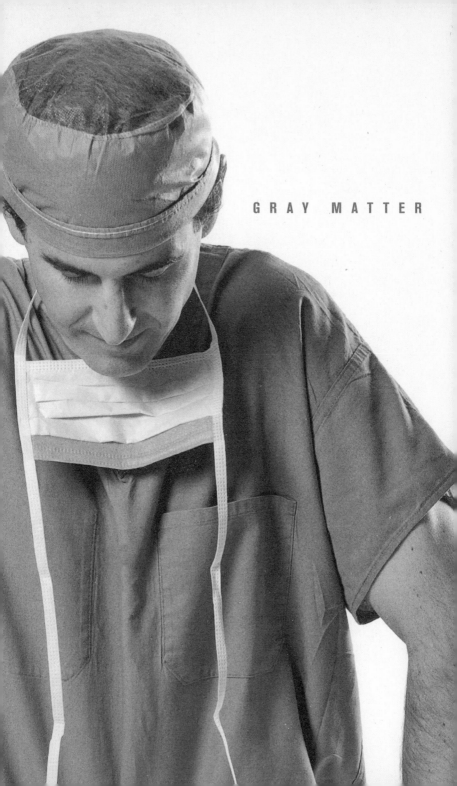

GRAY MATTER

GRAY
MATTER

a neurosurgeon discovers the power of prayer . . . one patient at a time

DAVID LEVY, MD
WITH JOEL KILPATRICK

Tyndale House Publishers, Inc.
Carol Stream, Illinois

Visit Tyndale's exciting Web site at www.tyndale.com.

TYNDALE and Tyndale's quill logo are registered trademarks of Tyndale House Publishers, Inc.

Gray Matter: A Neurosurgeon Discovers the Power of Prayer . . . One Patient at a Time

Copyright © 2011 by David Levy and Joel Kilpatrick. All rights reserved.

Cover and interior photographs copyright © by Tyndale House Publishers, Inc. All rights reserved.

Designed by Mark Anthony Lane II

Published in association with the literary agency of WordServe Literary Group, Ltd., 10152 S. Knoll Circle, Highlands Ranch, CO 80130.

Scripture quotations are taken from the *Holy Bible*, New Living Translation, copyright © 1996, 2004, 2007 by Tyndale House Foundation. Used by permission of Tyndale House Publishers, Inc., Carol Stream, Illinois 60188. All rights reserved.

Library of Congress Cataloging-in-Publication Data

Levy, David (David I.)
    Gray matter : a neurosurgeon discovers the power of prayer . . . one patient at a time / David Levy with Joel Kilpatrick.
        p. cm.
    Includes bibliographical references.
    ISBN 978-1-4143-3975-7 (sc)
    1. Medicine—Religious aspects—Christianity. 2. Nervous system—Surgery
3. Prayer—Christianity. I. Kilpatrick, Joel. II. Title.
    BT732.L48 2010
    261.5´61—dc22   2010050691

Printed in the United States of America

17   16   15   14   13   12   11
 7   6   5   4   3   2   1

This book is dedicated to my father, Isaac Levy, who passed away in 2001. Dad, you were a man of integrity and hard work, on whose shoulders I now stand. You demonstrated courage in the face of adversity, and only now do I realize all that you gave me. After we reconciled in 1997, I asked you to give me a father's blessing. You wrote, "That you may be happy in your work and in your endeavors . . . and that you continue growing." This book is the fulfillment of that blessing. I know that we will meet again, and when we do, we will have much to celebrate.

Contents

Acknowledgments

I WOULD LIKE TO THANK talented writer Joel Kilpatrick, who took my dream and made it a reality; Tyndale House acquisition editor Carol Traver, whose advice and expertise guided the project smoothly from start to finish, and editor Cara Peterson, whose insight and editorial skills proved invaluable; and Greg Johnson, my agent, who played an important part in this process.

I wish to extend my heartfelt thanks to those others who made valuable suggestions or contributions to the manuscript, in alphabetical order: Donald Adema, D.O.; SooHo Choi, M.D.; David and Anne Cliffe; Roberto Cueva, M.D., F.A.C.S.; Diane DePaul; Debbie Foreman; Jim Foreman, L.M.F.T.; Clem Hoffman, M.D.; Sandra Langley; Katherine Levy; Vera Levy; Doreen Hung Mar, M.D.; Merrill Nanigian; Mary Ann Nguyen-Kwok; William Rambo, M.D.; Scott Ricketts; Nguyen-Thi Robinson, M.D.; Natalie Rodriguez, M.D.; Mark Slomka; Jamie Wilson; Jordan Ziegler, M.D.

CHAPTER I

RISK FACTORS

MARIA, THE WELL-DRESSED BUSINESSWOMAN sitting in my office, had a brain aneurysm. One of the blood vessels in her brain had weakened, causing the vessel wall to balloon out in one place like a snake that has swallowed an egg. From the size and irregular shape of the aneurysm I had concluded that if not dealt with relatively quickly it might burst and kill her.

She was employed in high-level management and looked the part: she wore a black suit and heels, and an attaché case that appeared to be full of paperwork, presentations, and binders rested on the chair next to her. It looked as if she might be here on a lunch break between important meetings. I half expected her to say something like, "I've got ten

1

minutes until my face-to-face with clients, Doc. Make it snappy." But I could see that this sudden and unexpected diagnosis was causing her concern—a brain aneurysm isn't exactly one of those things you put on your calendar and schedule into your life.

It was our first meeting. She had been referred to me a week earlier by the neurologist who had picked up on the aneurysm, an unexpected "catch" that might very well save Maria's life. Many brain problems don't announce themselves. Aneurysms, notoriously, give no warning; they hide in the brain until one day, when the blood pressure proves too great for the strength of the artery wall, they rupture and bleed, causing a tremendous headache, loss of consciousness—and eventual death. Sometimes, in the fortunate cases, the aneurysm will push against a nerve or brain structure and prompt some odd symptoms that might alert someone before a catastrophic rupture. In Maria's case, there hadn't even been a suspicion of an aneurysm. The MRI scan had been ordered for a completely different, minor concern. But like a video security system that happens to catch images of a wanted killer lurking in the background, the scan had detected this menace inside her skull.

My job was to fix it before it could do any real damage.

If you have a brain aneurysm less than seven millimeters in size, a quarter inch in diameter, the chance of it bleeding is relatively low, less than 2 percent per year. That means the chance of it not bleeding is greater than 98 percent every year, which is not a large risk. However, if it does bleed, the risk of death is high—30 percent of those whose aneurysms burst don't even reach the hospital alive. They die from the trauma of blood flooding the skull and having nowhere to exit. Of those who make it to the hospital, 30 percent end up with a major cognitive deficit of some sort, losing their ability to talk or walk or recall information or even recognize loved ones. They are not able to resume their previous lifestyles. These are the kinds of facts I have to lay out for patients when discussing whether or not to treat them. I have to tell them whether I think that aneurysm or other malformation we see on the scan has a good chance of bursting or harming them and, if so, how to fix it before it does.

As for Maria, I felt she had no choice. The nine-millimeter aneurysm had multiple weak spots, or "daughter sacks," and was large, unstable, and unpredictable. It had to be treated.

We sat across from each other in my exam room at the San Diego hospital where I practice. The room is nothing special, your typical ten-by-ten medical box with a sink, cabinet, and window looking out on the trees in the parking lot. Nothing about it bespeaks comfort. Only my own nature photography hanging on the walls sets it apart from any other room in any other medical facility in America. Lining one wall are seats for the patient and family, though there was nobody here today but Maria and me. Just off to one side is a rolling computer stand into which I enter data and can review a patient's scans. Now I turned the computer screen around and showed Maria a 3-D rotational picture of the aneurysm from the CT angiogram. The multilobed, balloon-shaped aneurysm arose from her smooth brain artery like a phantom from a drainpipe.

"Let me lay out how I would approach this technically," I said. On the wall behind me was a whiteboard on which I drew a picture of her aneurysm and then detailed the treatment plan, to help her understand what would be taking place inside her skull while she was asleep. After a moment, I swiveled gently away from the board to face her. This was an important moment for both of us. In spite of her professional demeanor, Maria was now giving all the visible signals of agitation: arms and legs held uncomfortably tight against her body, eyes and facial muscles tense and alert. She kept making quick motions with her head and unconscious repetitive movements with her fingers. If she was trying to hold the anxiety in, it wasn't working; the tension was spilling out. Maria seemed to be wondering if her life, so full of the things she had hoped and planned for, was coming to an end. It was as if someone had slammed on the brakes and turned sharply into a blind alley called brain surgery.

As the neurosurgeon walking her through this difficult news, I had a complex set of tasks to perform. I had to ease her mind about the upcoming procedure, giving her the confidence that it could be successful and that she could come out of it without any loss of function. I also had to be honest with her about the level of risk it involved—of blindness, coma, paralysis, or death—so that she could properly set her own expectations and those of her family. We could not avoid the possibility that, as with any surgery in so delicate an area, things could go terribly wrong. I had to convey all this in a calm, honest, and straightforward way—to someone who really didn't want to hear it.

So much of a doctor's job is in not just diagnosis but in demeanor and presentation as well—the way you come across as you speak, the way you comport yourself, the way you relate to patients. Are your eyes steady, or are they shifty? Do you look into their eyes or over their shoulders or around the room? What does this subtly tell them about their prognosis? What can they read into your body language, your hand motions, your almost imperceptible movements of facial muscles, your ease or lack of ease, and your willingness to engage with them as persons, not just medical problems? Pre-surgical consultation is a dance. You have to practice it, becoming light on your feet and making the right moves in sequence, for it to seem graceful to you and to your patients. Fortunately, I have a calm manner that seems to set people at ease. Still, it takes a great deal of experience to make bedside manner seem effortless, and ultimately that is what you want to achieve: a sense of peace and confidence in spite of a bad diagnosis.

I explained the risks and benefits of intervention, and the risks and benefits of doing nothing. She nodded and followed along, taking it all in. As she looked at me, her eyes pleading for good news, I knew she was waiting for me to tell her that there was a pill or an easy treatment—something quick and painless that would solve her problem. Most patients believe, or at least hope, that a doctor can do anything. We are the modern medical high priests, called upon in almost spiritual fashion to rid people of the inconveniences of illness and to heal on demand. At least, that's how people treat us and how, especially in my field of neurosurgery, we often want to be treated. But I had made a decision to give up the role of high priest, even if I still looked like one in my white coat and light blue scrubs—the standard, intimidating outfit that helps to signal the surgeon's separation from and, technically speaking, superiority to the people around us. Yes, I am a highly trained medical professional, but I am not my patients' ultimate healer, and I certainly am not their god. I believe that position is already taken.

I glanced over her scans one more time, knowing full well that, with her, there was only one way to go.

"Maria, I recommend we take care of that aneurysm," I said. "It is the type we call a berry aneurysm because it has a small 'neck' holding it to the parent vessel. The aneurysm itself is round like a berry. Unfortunately, this kind has thin walls, and your thin walls have thinner walls called 'daughter sacks,' which I believe make it more likely to burst."

She didn't even exhale when I said this. It was as though she were holding her breath, waiting for the good part. She wanted me to tell her that she would be fine, but I could not promise that. Looking at this woman in the prime of her life and career, I was struck yet again by the fact that people with nothing outwardly wrong can have a ticking time bomb inside their heads.

I felt compassion and a familiar sense of peace. It would be tricky, but I had the skills to help her, and I loved using those skills; we were going to mend this thing so she could get on with the rest of her life. I wanted nothing more than to help put this incident firmly in her past. Ideally, she wouldn't see the inside of a hospital again until we did follow-up scans several months later to monitor her progress. Unlike other relationships, most surgeon-patient relationships should be temporary. We come together, solve the problem, and then go our separate ways.

"Can it wait?" she finally asked.

Statistically, it could; an aneurysm of that size had been there a long time. But those who have been in the business long enough have seen people bleed before they can get into surgery.

"If your aneurysm were perfectly round or smaller, I would have no problem waiting," I said. "We could wait a month—but I don't feel good about the size and shape."

She nodded slightly. "Then I guess that's what I have to do," she said. "I'm sure I'll have more questions when I've had a chance to digest this and research it a little more, and after I tell my family."

We both sat quietly as she considered again what I had said. After a moment, I leaned forward slightly and did what had become customary for me, something that I had never seen another doctor do, something that in a single moment stripped me of any semblance of godlike status.

"I know that I have given you a lot to think about. Would it be okay if I said a prayer with you?" I asked in a tone that made it safe for her to say no if she wished. I had asked earlier about her spiritual history and learned that her parents were Catholic but that she did not attend services.

She tilted her head to one side and looked at me curiously, as if reading a financial report she didn't understand. She relaxed slightly and nodded.

"Uh, okay," she said, a little confused. "Fine."

I slid my rolling chair over to her and slowly reached out my hand. As surprised as she was, she instinctively reached out with both of her hands and grabbed it as if grabbing a lifeline. I bowed my head to give her privacy. Then I began to pray.

"God, thank you for Maria and for allowing us to find this problem," I said. "This is a surprise to us but no surprise to you. I am asking that this aneurysm not cause her any problems until we can fix it. Please give her peace and good sleep leading up to this surgery. God, we are asking you for success for this surgery. Give her the sense that you are with her. In Jesus' name, Amen."

I opened my eyes after the short prayer. Maria's chin was on her chest and she was crying softly. Tears had made water marks on her skirt. Peace seemed to blanket her, and she was tranquil and centered, like a visitor in a church or other sacred place. Gone were the extraneous movements born of high stress. She breathed deeply and seemed to exhale the concerns that had nearly overtaken her. This sudden change might have surprised me if I hadn't seen it happen so many times with so many other people.

After a few moments she looked up at me. Tears were

blending with her mascara and running down her cheeks in gray streaks. She nodded her affirmation of the prayer and dabbed her nose with a tissue that I handed her from the box I keep on my computer stand.

"Thank you, Dr. Levy," she said with a sparkle in her eyes that spoke of calm and hope. "I've never prayed with a doctor before."

I smiled. I'd heard that many times. This simple act had done what no conversation, no psychological analysis, no recitation of the medical facts had ever done, in my experience. She had received something no insurance company, medical provider, surgeon, or drug could offer: confidence and peace from a simple prayer. And even, I believe, a welcome touch from God.

Maria's surgery went flawlessly—until the very end. Then a tear in the aneurysm caused blood to flow into the spaces of her brain with every heartbeat. I feared the worst; we might not be able to save her.

With my crew waiting for instructions, I called for the specific tools I would need to repair the breach. Everything seemed to happen in slow motion, and I felt my frustration rise. There is nothing surgeons hate more than surprises, especially the kind that could rob this family of a wife and mother.

I guided my instruments up the carotid artery just below the bleeding aneurysm and tried another method to stop the bleeding from the potentially fatal tear in the vessel wall. After five minutes of intensely focused work, I injected dye to see if I had succeeded. My heart sank as I watched the screen and saw the dye leak from the top of the aneurysm as she continued to bleed. She had been bleeding into the brain for more than five minutes. Would she survive? And if she did, what would she be like?

It took several more minutes of delicate, painstaking work and periods of agonizing waiting, but finally the bleeding stopped. It took another hour to determine that Maria would survive the bleed and had not suffered a major stroke; she was moving her arms and legs and was talking. As she went into the intensive care unit and continued to improve over the next few days, I thanked God for answering the prayer that Maria and I had prayed together in my exam room. I believe it made the difference for Maria—and for me.

Because in neurosurgery, you never know what might happen.

• • •

I have no way of knowing exactly how many nurses, doctors, surgeons, or even other neurosurgeons take the spiritual lives of their patients seriously or pray with their patients as I do. It's certainly not a subject that comes up at medical conferences or with coworkers in the elevator or hospital cafeteria. In fact, if spirituality is not introduced in a way that honors the patient and his or her faith, it can lead to ostracism by the medical community or worse—discipline of some kind. The role of prayer in health care is itself a gray matter.

Yet both doctors and patients seem to recognize that some crucial component of patient care is often missing. Though spirituality is almost completely absent from medical interactions, a large majority (75 percent) of more than a thousand physicians surveyed agree that religion and spirituality are important in helping patients cope and in giving them a positive state of mind.[1]

Patients, too, place a high value on religion and spirituality, particularly in the midst of an illness. In one study, 82 percent of 124 consecutive ophthalmology patients at Johns Hopkins University said prayer was important to their sense of well-being.[2]

As I have addressed patients' spirituality and made prayer a regular part of my patient interactions, the response has been impressive. I have seen lives brought to a level of spiritual, emotional, and physical health that my patients had never enjoyed before. In the process, I have learned two important things: that there is a limit to what I can do as a highly trained and experienced surgeon and that there is no limit to what God can do to touch a person emotionally and spiritually, not just physically.

My goal as a professional is to use my skills and knowledge to help people have the best lives possible, for as long as possible. This includes emotional as well as physical health, because the two are interrelated. Emotions can create health or cause disease, and spiritual health affects emotional health. Laughter and joy are known to restore and encourage health, while bitterness and resentment promote disease.

Forgiveness has well-documented health benefits. One's concept of God can cause ongoing joy or ongoing anxiety. These, issues are not incidental but are central to health.[3]

The responsible thing for a doctor to do is to give patients the opportunity to make healthy choices in all areas of life.

• • •

As a neurosurgeon, I see a lot of tough cases. I am at the end of a chain of doctors that begins, usually, with primary care or emergency room physicians. Patients may start the journey toward neurosurgery because of minor problems such as headaches, dizziness, or tingling sensations that prompt them to go to the emergency room or see their primary care physicians. Some are sent to a neurologist, who orders an MRI scan.

Just to be clear, neurologists do not operate on the body; neurosurgeons do. Neurologists are the Ansel Adamses of the brain world, taking pictures of the brain and nervous system with various types of equipment—EEGs, EMGs, MRIs, and so on—to try to pinpoint a problem. Their challenge is to diagnose and treat symptoms nobody else can figure out. They gather a myriad of symptoms, bundle them together, and label them with a diagnosis. Maybe those symptoms point to Parkinson's disease, multiple sclerosis, or one of the other neurological diseases that have a specific set of symptoms. Or maybe the symptoms form a random collection that doesn't tell you much of anything. In many cases the symptoms are caused by stress and anxiety. Much of the time nobody really knows why someone has a tingling arm, persistent headaches, or a "weird feeling" in some part of his or her body. Neurologists often have to tell patients, "I can't find anything to explain your symptoms." After all, most people with symptoms such as headaches, dizziness, or tingling do not have a brain aneurysm. Neurologists try to figure out who actually has disease. They have a difficult job.

The MRI scans neurologists order often prove invaluable because they can reveal an aneurysm or other malformation in the brain that nobody knew was there and that usually has nothing to do with the symptoms. We call this an incidental finding, and it is one of the reasons patients are redirected to me. They usually have small bumps on the vessels that are of no consequence. Occasionally—as in Maria's case—they are life-threatening problems.

I operate on the brain. If surgery is necessary—on a tumor, an aneurysm, a knot of malformed vessels, or something else—there are a few ways to go into the head to solve the problem. Open surgery enters in the "traditional" way: cutting a hole in the skull to reveal the melon-sized gray matter that functions as the repository of our memories, habits, knowledge, personalities, and everything else that make human life what it is. In the case of aneurysms, most of which are on the base of the brain between the lobes, open surgery involves peeling the lobes apart to work on the vessels. For aneurysm surgery, we must operate while constantly looking through a large, suspended microscope that is wheeled into position over the patient, a transparent sterile covering allowing it to be close to the open brain. I always enjoy that first look, when the *dura mater*—Latin for "tough mother," the leathery covering inside the skull—is pulled back and the glistening surface of the brain is exposed. It is like putting on a diving mask and looking beneath the surface of the water at a coral reef: a whole new world opens up, and I become completely absorbed by it. The microscope illuminates and magnifies the brain's awe-inspiring beauty, and the focus control brings it into sharp detail under powerful light. Against a nearly white background run arteries like red vines, branching into smaller arterioles and coursing through the sulci and gyri—the peaks and valleys of the cortex, the undulating surface of the brain.

People often ask me what it's like to operate on the brain, to look at it, touch it, and mend it. I tell them that working directly on the brain is simultaneously challenging and invigorating. The vessels—the arteries and veins—glisten and pulsate beautifully. The architecture of the brain itself and the vascular system that supplies it with blood and oxygen are staggeringly complex—far more complex than any spacecraft, supercomputer, or anything else built by human hands. The brain is the command center of the body. Everything we need—from basic body functions to the creation of art and music, speech and complex technology, love and every human endeavor—is contained in this elegant and relatively tiny package. To repair its vessels, to restore blood flow to the command center, is amazing. It is exhilarating to work around something so vital. This is the human body's most valuable real estate. Working in that neighborhood is one of the highest privileges I have.

I started out, like other neurosurgeons, doing open neurosurgery—drilling off a piece of the skull, putting my hands and instruments inside the brain, repairing the problem, and putting the skull piece back on. Later, I began to specialize in endovascular ("inside the vessels") work, which I could see was the future of the field. Because many problems in the brain occur in the vessels (the arteries and veins), technology increasingly allows us to treat them without drilling open the skull. We can insert our instruments into the femoral artery (in the leg) and travel three feet "north" into the brain itself. This type of surgery is less invasive. No cutting bone or opening someone's head. Most people like that idea.

There is nothing routine about going inside the brain, though, no matter which direction you're coming from. Endovascular neurosurgery is still difficult and dangerous. In fact, it is one of the most dangerous of all the specialties of neurosurgery, because anytime you're dealing with a damaged vessel, as in the case of an aneurysm, you know that the vessel wall has been injured or compromised. Sometimes any touch, any manipulation, can cause a damaged vessel to rupture and fill the brain with blood.

Every parent knows that head wounds bleed profusely. What turn out to be minor cuts appear at first to be massive gashes that somehow produce copious amounts of blood. That is also true within the head. The brain is a blood hog.

A measure of its importance is that, although the brain represents only 2 percent of total body weight, it receives 15 percent of the body's blood supply.

The brain's high demand for blood and oxygen, along with its lack of appreciable energy reserves, makes it uniquely susceptible to disruptions of the blood supply. When an aneurysm ruptures during open surgery, the blood streams out so freely and quickly that the operating field is flooded, making it difficult to see what you're doing. A straightforward procedure suddenly takes on the character of fixing a leaky pipe under muddy water: stopping the flow is not easy.

When you're operating on other parts of the body, you can clip vessels here and there to stop the blood flow and clear up your field without much consequence. However, in the brain you have to be exponentially more careful. This is a high-rent district, the information headquarters for the patient's entire life. There is no backup system. When the blood flows, you can't start blindly putting clips on whatever is nearby, because you might injure a vessel or nerve that allows the patient to sing, dance, swallow, read, talk, or recognize his or her grandchildren. The brain is a minefield of wonders, and you must move carefully. A sudden hemorrhage might obscure your vision and invite rash movements to stop it, but it is easy to make a bad situation worse. Even small movements of fingers and instruments can have big consequences, so neurosurgeons must develop a finely honed technical ability. They must also know where the bleeding problems are likely to happen and how to stop them.

I was fortunate to train under some of the finest neuro-surgeons in the world and have had a successful practice for more than fifteen years, but it is still a challenge to keep calm while adrenaline is pumping into my own bloodstream during a complicated surgery. With stroke or death looming large, controlling my own fear and rising panic becomes a learned skill. When things are going badly in neurosurgery, the potential loss is tremendous. I promise you, the neuro-surgeon feels it. Everyone else in the operating room can go home and sleep well after another day of work, but I often lie awake wondering what I should have done differently. In a sense, surgeons work utterly alone.

The complexity and challenge of the brain contribute, at least for me, to the great satisfaction of operating on it, but that comes with great stress and, at times, frustration. Even if you do the procedure technically perfectly, you can still end up with a bad result—a ruined life, a mental deficit, an erased memory. Unexpected things happen. Operating on the brain is a high-wire act that rarely offers you a safety net.

That sense of challenge is also a major reason that I pray—not because I lack confidence but because I am realistic about what I am able to do and confident about what God is able to do. Surgery can treat the immediate problem, but much more is involved in healing than just this physical aspect. Surgery is reactive, not proactive. Surgical outcomes are never com-pletely predictable. Some technically perfect procedures result in stroke or death for patients, while some potentially cata-strophic bleeds in the brain result in no loss of function at all.

Most surgeons chalk this up to fate, chance, or luck ("better lucky than good") because we cannot explain it, but I am convinced that there is much more at work than just "chance." I believe God wants to be involved—and will be, if we ask him.

This book tells the story of how I, a practicing neurosurgeon, began to address the spiritual and emotional aspects of health and to pray with the people I operate on. My journey to combining medicine and faith did not start easily. At first, I was not graceful or confident about it. I made some people uncomfortable. I'm reminded of the old bit of wisdom that if you want to do something well, you have to be willing to do it poorly at first. I began with no road map for praying with patients. This wasn't the kind of stuff we were taught in medical school or during residency. Even so, over time prayer worked into my normal routine and became natural. It made things better. I believe it changed outcomes.

Does everyone I pray for get better? No, and that is frustrating. I'm still waiting to receive that magic wand doctors are supposed to receive with their licenses to practice medicine. But I have seen many positive results from prayer, and I'm convinced they go beyond any physical or psychological explanation. Not only have people's brains been healed, but many people have been released from shackles of bitterness, anger, and resentment, which can be the root cause of serious physical problems. I have discovered that God sees the whole person, not just the particular problem that is flaring up in his or her head. Patients generally appreciate being seen as more than their medical problems.

I have been in this profession for a good number of years and am intimately familiar with most of the new techniques, procedures, medical devices, and drugs hitting the market. Many of them are ingenious, and I use them regularly in my practice. I have consulted for several companies to develop better devices and have traveled the world teaching others to use them. I admire and am grateful for modern medical technology. But though technology can prolong a life or reduce pain, it cannot always make life better.

My experiences have convinced me that spirituality is a crucial element to the well-being of a person as a whole; moreover, if we let him, God can do powerful, supernatural things in our everyday lives. That's why I began inviting God into my consultations, exams, and surgeries. Many would be surprised that a neurosurgeon—a man of science, logic, and human progress—would be such a strong believer in God and divine intervention. Yet the experience has been nothing short of phenomenal.

CHAPTER 2

HOW I BEGAN PRAYING WITH PATIENTS

It was decision time.

My heart was pounding as I climbed the back stairs at the hospital and entered the pre-operative area, the large room through which all patients pass on their way to surgery. Pre-op has the feel of a busy port: nurses, anesthesiologists, and doctors rush here and there holding charts and IV bags, pushing carts, carrying syringes and vials of medicine. Machines beep, dozens of worried family conversations mingle, televisions chatter, and everywhere you look are gurneys gliding by with patients on their way to surgery. It's a scene that normally fills me with confidence and energy. I am rarely nervous before surgery and am typically the portrait of the calm and self-assured neuro-surgeon. Even the smells of the hospital—rubbing alcohol, latex, sterilized steel and plastic—trigger feelings of cool control in me before I reach the patient. This is my arena, my playing field.

But today I was terrified.

I had made up my mind to pray with a patient for the first time. Not only had I never done that before, I had never even seen it done by anyone in the medical profession. Ours is mostly a faithless occupation where spiritual matters are kept firmly outside the boundaries in which we function. For most doctors, faith and feelings are something for the chaplains, nurses, or family to deal with, like a messy or irri-tating side effect or even a weakness in the patient. Those of us paid to operate on the body, to make physical things right, to restore life are supposed to be above spirituality somehow. We are surgeons and scientists, people of facts and high train-ing and confidence that can sometimes border on (or bound boldly into) arrogance. But I could no longer deny what I felt God had been encouraging me to do, even though it seemed unthinkable. With one decision I was about to put my reputation, my professional relationships, even my career on the line.

Like most doctors, I had always made a habit of speak-ing with each patient before surgery. Traditionally this serves several purposes. First, it verifies that this, indeed, is the person you're supposed to be operating on, and not some guy down the hall. People love telling stories about doctors removing the wrong organ or amputating the wrong limb, though these incidents are very rare. To avoid giving those stories any more credence and to avoid ruining or complicating someone's life with a wrong procedure, I talk face-to-face with patients on the day of surgery. Second, this visit assures that we are all—surgeon, patient, family—on the same page about what we are doing, the risks involved, and what we want the outcome to be. If someone, maybe a family member, has not understood the risks fully up to now, this is the time to make them clear. Third, it gives the patient and family confidence in me as a surgeon. If the doctor exudes confidence, they have confidence too. That's good for morale and, arguably, for outcomes. This brings up the last and usually unstated reason many doctors, and certainly I, have often enjoyed meeting with patients in pre-op: it gives us a sense of accomplishment. There we stand in our white coats and scrubs at the foot of the bed, about to work on a person's brain with tiny, expensive medical instruments while he or she is unconscious. We are entrusted with people's very lives. That is why we hold an exalted place in society, why we are paid well. It is the apex of all we have worked to achieve.

But this day was entirely different for me. Pre-op was as busy as ever when I walked into Mrs. Jones's area. She was lying on her gurney, the rolling stretcher that would transport her to surgery. The attending nurse looked up as I entered. If you've ever been in surgery or attended someone about to undergo it, you may already know that in pre-op there are not rooms as such, but bays separated by thin curtains hanging from shower-style ceiling tracks. You can hear everything that's going on in the neighboring bay, including the blather from the televisions hanging from the ceiling in each stall and all but the quietest conversations. Privacy is minimal and mostly imagined.

"Good morning. How are you today?" I asked Mrs. Jones as I stood next to her gurney.

"A little nervous, I guess," she said, her smile clearly tinged with anxiety. Her two young adult daughters stood nearby, saying nothing and observing me intently, arms folded. One of them smiled faintly in my direction.

I began to go through the brief presentation I give to patients on their way to surgery, reviewing her case, the possible outcomes from the procedure, and our desired outcome. Yet inside my chest, my heart was hammering so hard that, at least in my ears, it competed with the general din of pre-op and the sound of my own voice. Now that I was here, in the room with an actual patient, the idea of introducing prayer and spiritual matters seemed far-fetched and even dangerous. There was no telling how Mrs. Jones or her daughters would react. I continued on, working hard to make sure my feelings weren't noticeable as I went over my notes with her one last time. As I spoke, Mrs. Jones nodded that she understood. Thankfully, she didn't seem to notice my inner agitation.

Strangely for a perfectionist like me, I had not thought about when or how I would add prayer to my routine. Somehow I figured I would do it on the fly or perhaps feel inspired at a certain moment to offer to pray. This lack of planning now struck me as a major mistake, like going onstage without ever looking at a script. I had checked her admission form and seen that her religion was listed as "Protestant." That gave me a bit of a safety net if I jumped off this cliff. She would at least be familiar with prayer. If I had seen "None," I might have canceled my plans. That would have been too much risk for my first time. I was also concerned that the nurse, who was still preparing Mrs. Jones for an intravenous drip, was not leaving. I had made a firm decision that I was not going to pray with anyone else around. To be honest, I was scared of letting anyone else in the hospital know what I was about to do. I would wait until I was alone with Mrs. Jones and her daughters. Only then would I perhaps be able to summon the courage to ask her.

"We've already talked about the risks of the operation," I continued. "You will have a small puncture site in the artery when we finish. I'll be going up into the brain to repair this aneurysm . . ."

As I spoke, I drew out the explanation and spoke more slowly than usual, hoping that in the meantime the nurse would leave so I could carry out my plan. But the nurse seemed in no hurry. She was well occupied with her checklist, taking Mrs. Jones's blood pressure and temperature, hooking her up to a vital signs monitor, and recording her medications. Nurses in pre-op always have checklists of tasks to carry out. The list can vary in content and length depending on the surgeon, the procedure, and the anesthesiologist. It usually includes such tasks as checking the patient's belongings, making sure the patient is not wearing false teeth, eyeglasses, or jewelry when he or she goes to surgery. They ask if the patient is pregnant, has had the flu recently, or is allergic to any medications. They might even draw blood for labwork or get an electrocardiogram (an EKG) to check for any problems with the heart before we put it under stress. Today, this nurse slowly moved from one task to another with no sign of finishing. I kept glancing over at her, waiting for her to wrap it up, but it almost seemed that she was working against me.

Mrs. Jones nodded after my presentation was finished. None of this was new to her, or to me. I tried to think of something else to say to extend the conversation. All I could come up with was the typical capper: "Do you have any more questions?"

I looked at her daughters hopefully. Doctors often hate getting questions in the rushed moments before surgery, but this time I was soliciting them as best I could with my open expression.

"How long will it take?" one daughter blessedly asked.

"That's a good question," I said, preparing to give a lengthy answer. I shot a brief look again at the nurse, who tapped obliviously on her keyboard, entering more data into Mrs. Jones's computer records. It was as if we were competing to see who could outlast the other.

When I had finished my explanation, managing to consume several minutes with a vague answer that explained the various factors preventing me from making a firm declaration about the surgery's duration, still the nurse was not finished. My heart was nearly in my throat now. In addition, I felt the distress of having failed to carry out my purpose to pray. But I now had no other reason to be in the room. If I overstayed, Mrs. Jones and her daughters would begin to wonder what was wrong.

I smiled with disappointed finality.

"Great. If there are no more questions, I'll see you after the procedure," I said.

"Thank you, Doctor," Mrs. Jones said. I turned to go and glimpsed the nurse slowly rubbing alcohol on Mrs. Jones's arm in preparation for the IV. I felt momentarily like ordering the nurse out of the room—I was, after all, the senior medical professional. I wouldn't even have to give an explanation. This action would have been too disruptive and unusual, though, and would call too much attention to what I was doing. Instead, I admitted defeat and ducked through the curtains. Frustrated, I stepped back into the main pre-op room.

In spite of being tempted to breeze out as I had so many times before, I decided not to give up. To buy time, I wandered slowly over to the central nurses' station, the vibrant hub of the pre-op area. I took in the computers, stacks of papers, charts, wheeled carts, long desks, cabinets full of records and various other administrative paraphernalia. Nurses came and went on their various assignments. I felt awkward being there without any clear purpose, but I had made up my mind—today was not going to be a normal day. I was going to at least ask Mrs. Jones if I could pray for her.

I would conquer my anxiety. Somehow, against all my fears and all practical obstacles, I was going to make it happen.

• • •

For years the idea of praying for patients before surgery had hounded me. I'm not even sure when it first occurred to me to try, but over time the feeling swelled from a ripple to a tidal wave. I had prayed privately during difficult moments at surgery, usually under my breath, as many doctors do. I had even prayed for cases in private, before surgery. But to pray audibly and in the presence of a patient was something very different. I had no point of reference for doing this and could not imagine what prayer would look like in a medical practice. At what point in the process would I bring up the patient's spiritual journey? Where would it happen? What would it look like? How would I initiate it? What would I say? The logistics escaped me. Textbooks never addressed it. Nobody I knew modeled it. For me, this was completely uncharted territory.

In all my training and in practice, I had never seen a physician pray for a patient or acknowledge God in any way, unless you count the "Oh God" muttered when bleeding shot out from a totally unexpected source or could not be stopped quickly during surgery. Surgeons are generally not, by nature or reputation, spiritual people. Even beyond their spirituality, or lack of it, surgeons pride themselves in being scientific, not touchy-feely. It is almost as if the medical training shapes us into the same mold, and when we receive our license, we also don new personalities that fit the standards of our breed. The surgeon's motto is "heal with steel." The subject of God or religion comes with a certain tension when it is merely brought up in the hospital, let alone associated with outcomes. Surgeons dislike the mystical. I felt that broaching the subject with patients would seem as bizarre to my colleagues as my bringing a crystal ball into the room and recommending that we all consult it before surgery.

To say that praying out loud with a patient before surgery would put me out on a limb is putting it too mildly. It would catapult me out of the tree.

•   •   •

During my many years of medical school, residency, fellowship training, and then out in practice, I have observed that many of my colleagues viewed people with religious beliefs as simpleminded. As for me, I was captivated by the power of surgery; compared to that power, faith seemed quaint at best, necessary only if there were no surgical options. When we had to delay surgery until a priest or rabbi arrived, we felt inconvenienced. When religious beliefs limited our options, such as the refusal of a blood transfusion on religious grounds, we saw it as a menace, a silly superstition.

In medical school we had talked a little about what was called the "art of medicine." This included the creativity to elicit the correct history, the insight to ask the right questions, and the meticulous attention to detail that would lead us to order the right test and thus lead us to the correct diagnosis. This method of diagnosis, which occasionally touched on areas of spirituality or emotion, was used much more in the days before CT and MRI scans. I had always approached this area of "study" with the idea that spirituality and medicine were weakly connected and could be explained by the placebo effect: if some people thought their faith would help them, then they would improve merely because they believed it. It was the same power I believed many alternative medicines had: the power of positive thinking.

As I began treating my own patients instead of hypothetical patients in a classroom, I began to see my own carefully honed surgical skills fail to produce the outcomes I expected. I had faith in surgery and had given many years of my life to acquiring the skills necessary to do the most difficult operations. I had thought that if I could do a procedure perfectly, I would get a perfect result every time. I was wrong.

It was out of the disappointment over bad outcomes—any bad outcomes—that I began to appreciate the connection between our physical and spiritual lives. I was growing in my knowledge of God and beginning to respect the spiritual world in my personal life. Though I still insisted that there was no place for it in the hospital, my opinion on that, too, slowly began to change. The line between the two areas blurred; my reasons for separating them began to crumble.

Empirical evidence confirms the connection. Studies have shown that approximately one in five patients (19 percent) want their physicians to pray with them on a routine office visit;[1] 29–48 percent of hospitalized patients want prayer from their physicians;[2] 40 percent of patients welcome physicians' exploring religious or spiritual issues with them; and only 7 percent do not believe in the power of prayer.[3] An article in one medical journal states, "A large proportion of published empirical data suggests that religious commitment may play a beneficial role in preventing mental and physical illness, improving how people cope with mental and physical illness and facilitating recovery from illness."[4] Another journal article concludes, "Over 35 systematic reviews have all concluded that in the vast majority of patients, the apparent benefits of intrinsic religious belief and practice outweigh the risks."[5]

I could no longer ignore my impulse to offer patients more than just physical care, when there was much more to them than their bodies.

Then the pivotal moment arrived. I found myself in a dentist's chair on a Saturday preparing to have a filling replaced. My dentist friend, who had come into the office on his day off just to do this procedure on me, had the novocaine syringe with the long needle in his hand. Like most surgeons, I hate having the needle or scalpel turned on me. I don't mind wielding it on others, but I'll go to great lengths to avoid being on the receiving end of a sharp point. My dentist friend sensed my apprehension, put his other hand on my shoulder, and said a short prayer asking God to guide his hands during the procedure. A sense of peace washed over me, and I relaxed. The needle didn't hurt as I had thought it would, the procedure went fine, and I went home feeling not just fixed but encouraged.

That experience confirmed the growing feeling in my heart that God wanted me to pray with my patients before surgery and transmit that same kind of peace to them. Still, I remained skeptical and opposed to the idea of prayer before surgery, having many good reasons to think it was a bad one. I reviewed these on my ride home:

To call on a higher power would be to admit weakness or lack of control. Prayer, I thought, would be seen as an admission that I was lacking in confidence, ease, or skill in the procedure I was about to perform. This was exactly the opposite of what any doctor wishes to convey to anyone else—patient, nurse, or colleague. It could very well alarm a patient at a critical moment and cause him or her to doubt my abilities.

Patients may be offended. How many of them would think I was trying to convert them or badger them with religion? Was it even appropriate in this context? It seemed to violate the professionalism inherent in good medicine. I didn't want to cause offense, and I didn't want any complaints.

If I prayed and things went badly, it could ruin patients' faith. What if that happened? Would it shake their faith or make it less likely that they would ever want to know God? Would they be angry with me or with God?

I still believed in the separation of the physical and the spiritual. Even though I was growing as a follower of Jesus, I was trained to respect the gulf between medicine and religion. Doctors are science based. Chaplains and certain alternative medicine practitioners are not, and they are therefore free to use anecdotal and unproven methods. They are also less respected by many because their training is less demanding. Only for them is prayer the "standard of care."

I would lose my reputation in the medical community. My colleagues simply would not accept or respect someone who introduced spiritual matters, or what they might term "superstition," into the practice of medicine. They would have more sympathy if I were to confess to alcoholism or mental illness or even attempt suicide. Appealing to a divine being would be akin to using incantations or good-luck charms. By praying—and relying on something other than science—I would be admitting that science did not have all the answers, and I would in effect be giving up my exalted position in the scientific community.

I wanted to be credited for my successes. I was trained to believe that success in surgery is always the result of applied knowledge and expert technical skills. I believed that the intellectual acumen needed to correctly diagnose a problem and the ability to technically execute a plan comprised the real healing power; I had worked diligently to obtain and apply this expertise. To suggest that knowledge and skills were inadequate would be to challenge not only my own sense of self-worth but the very way in which medicine is practiced.

I was introducing an unnecessary variable. Performing surgery is about controlling variables—that is, minimizing the number of unquantifiable risks. The fewer the variables, the better. Prayer would introduce an unnecessary variable into an already stressful and difficult situation. It would create a condition in which I didn't know what might happen or whether it would upset the patient or the family.

In addition to these reasons, one other thing disconcerted me a great deal: *Praying would alter the typical doctor-patient relationship.* That relationship usually puts the surgeon in the superior position. Surgery is the doctor's show to run. The patient is often a passive participant, not a partner. I am seen as the one with all the answers. Prayer would make patients equal partners with me. In fact, I would need to ask permission to pray. This didn't feel familiar to me. They were in the position of asking me for my services; would I now ask them for permission to pray? Would that be desirable? Would it even be proper? Would I lose respect? Or worse?

In truth, the doctor-patient relationship is based on something more than hierarchy—it's at least partially based on fear. Doctors fear being sued; patients fear a bad outcome. This is the overriding dynamic of the relationship, especially when it involves a high-risk surgery, which includes every brain surgery. Because of the fear of being sued, doctors are very careful not to let their humanity turn into any sort of vulnerability. The questions in the back, or front, of their minds are always, How could this relationship go bad? What might turn this happy scene into a lawsuit? The questions in patients' minds are, The doctor seems nice, but is he or she competent? What if something goes wrong? What will happen to me?

Being sued is one of the few possibilities that make doctors feel vulnerable. It is the worst possible scenario for a medical professional, because it means someone has broken through the protective barrier of your life and threatens your personal and professional well-being. A patient is calling into question the thing that sits at the core of your self-image—your competence. This person is accusing you of something that you never intended to happen and perhaps wasn't even your fault. Once you've been through that, the pain lingers for a long time, so to protect yourself, you start to worry only about dotting the *i*'s and crossing the *t*'s. It's no longer entirely about a patient's health or well-being; it is also about getting you, the doctor, through the procedure with the best possible result and without a lawsuit. In that sense, you are united in purpose with the patient, but for many physicians, a significant motivation is self-preservation—to avoid becoming personally or professionally vulnerable to the patient.

It is easy to understand the vulnerability of the patients. They long to hear good news, and I can sense that longing as soon as I walk into the room. Most doctors I know try to be upbeat and friendly, and this, I think, is because doctors have incredible power to impart feelings—confidence or anxiety, peace or stress. I often want to say with a big smile, "This is going to go perfectly," because that is what patients want to hear to put them at ease. But it goes both ways: surgeons can be affected by the feelings of their patients, too. In this way, the dynamic of fear also occasionally works against successful outcomes.

When patients or family members demonstrate excessive fear, this can affect a surgeon's mood. Surgeons cannot share that fear of failure because it is an affront to their profession-alism and (if they accept the affront) it can potentially affect the success of a surgery. They may regard a patient's fear as a challenge to perform flawlessly. Surgeons are perfection-ists, but this inevitably heightens their anxiety going into a procedure. This added stress doesn't lead to better results. In fact, when a demanding patient wants to be treated like a VIP, the chance of an unforeseen problem is usually higher. I wish it weren't so.

The first thing that comes to my mind when surgery starts going badly is, *This person may die or be debilitated, and I am responsible. How will the family react?* I know what it's like to try to control unexpected bleeding while at the same time imagining what it will be like to explain to the family that things didn't go well and that the patient—their mother, father, son, daughter, or friend—will never be the same person they had known before. It is mental and physi-cal torment.

Prayer would redefine the kind of doctor-patient relation-ship I had grown comfortable with. It would strike down this idea that I was a demigod. It would make me vulnerable in a way I had never been vulnerable with a patient before. Certainly, I wouldn't be as vulnerable as someone who is asleep while undergoing an operation, but I would be vulnerable in sharing who I am as a person and in relinquishing the surgeon's detachment and mystique. I would be deliberately climbing down from the pedestal and admitting my humanity. And in medicine, as in the rest of life, vulnerability is dangerous.

Despite all my apprehension about prayer's role, I felt that to be authentic I needed to somehow make it part of my patient interactions. I felt there was something sorely missing there. I was doing one of the most technically difficult and highest paid jobs in the world, but somehow I knew there was more. Up until now I had been doing only what I was trained to do: extending life and relieving pain, worry, or inconvenience. What about improving life quality by helping people to be more joyful, loving, and kind? Was it possible for me as a neurosurgeon to help them have a different kind of life, to help them examine themselves and make a course correction, and to do so in a way that would not be offensive? Or could I only extend their lives on their current trajectories?

Through all my questions and doubts I felt an inner voice saying to me, "If you are worried about being misunderstood, I can promise you that you will be. Jesus was. But you still need to do the right thing."

After practicing neurosurgery for seven years, I knew that praying for a patient before surgery was the right thing to do, and I decided to ask the next patient, regardless of what might happen.

• • •

That opportunity arrived the very next week with Mrs. Jones. I had gone into her pre-op room with the intention of praying, but in the presence of that powerful and intimidating nurse, I had retreated and been forced to reformulate my approach.

Fear was still governing my decisions. *Couldn't I just pray silently for her?* I thought. *Maybe I'll pray with the next one.*

I leaned against the desk at the nurses' station, feeling awkward at being there and riffling through papers on my clipboard as if they were of great importance. Nurses, patients, and patients' families passed by me. I kept my head down and my eye surreptitiously on Mrs. Jones's gurney, watching for the nurse to leave. For some reason her area and the adjacent bays were a hive of nurse activity. It looked like a receiving line in there. The longer I waited, the more nervous I felt—more nervous, in fact, than I was before any surgery that I could remember. During surgery I am in my comfort zone; here, I was way outside. I, the most highly trained person in the room, felt intimidated by everyone else in pre-op.

Why are so many nurses visiting Mrs. Jones? I thought, growing perturbed. This was a fairly straightforward procedure. What else could there possibly be for them to do?

I looked back down and pretended to be reviewing the chart for as long as this charade seemed to hold. There was little to read: my history from the week before and her blood tests. I carefully examined some of the fine print at the bottom of the page. Then I walked over to the phone sitting on the counter and made some calls. I checked my home voice mail. I checked my office messages. I tried to think of who else I might call—old friends, anybody—but nobody was awake this early. Then I pretended to be on a call, but that lasted only until the dead line turned into an annoying beep, and I had to hang up. The nurses were still busy in Mrs. Jones's room, checking that her belongings were safely stowed under her bed, entering more data into the bedside computer. *Maybe they're training a newbie nurse*, I thought. But I realized if I didn't act soon, the transportation team would come to get Mrs. Jones and take her to the procedure room. Patients don't stay long in pre-op—usually less than ninety minutes. The idea is not to park people there at length but to move them on to the main event.

I was about to miss my chance.

Then suddenly, the nurse left. I stood up and began to walk over. I scrutinized the curtained bays next to hers as well, because I had resolved not to pray if a nurse was on either side of the curtain. Could it be? It was true: Mrs. Jones was alone with her two daughters. The two adjoining bays were empty except for patients. Perfect. I headed over, feeling a surge of renewed confidence.

Before I could get there, the anesthesiologist and nurse anesthetist arrived. I smiled at them, stopped short—then redirected my steps back to the nurses' station. There was no way I was praying in front of an anesthesiologist. I walked over to a sink and washed my hands for the third or fourth time. I tried to find an out-of-the-way place to stand where I wouldn't be too conspicuous to the nurses, who must have been wondering what a doctor was doing hanging around their turf.

How strange, I thought. It was as if I were casing her room, waiting to commit a crime.

After an achingly long time, the anesthesiologist and nurse anesthetist left. I saw no transport team approaching. The nurses had gone to other rooms. This was my final opportunity. I darted over, trying to seize the territory before anyone else could. I glanced at the patients on both sides, uncomfortable with the fact that they might hear me. For once I was happy that their television volumes were loud enough to possibly obscure my voice. I cringed as I noticed the thin curtains separating us.

Mrs. Jones was sitting up on the gurney with an IV in her arm, looking as relaxed as could be expected before such a major surgery. Her daughters were seated by the bed. The overhead fluorescent lights seemed to drain all faces of color. When they saw me, they stood up to receive whatever news I had.

Only then did I realize that I had not even thought of how I would introduce the subject, let alone what I would say in the prayer. I assumed it would be simple and obvious. Maybe I had thought that too much planning wasn't desirable when it came to spiritual things. Now my mouth felt like sand; my heart raced as if I'd just been injected with epinephrine. Gone was the good-natured confidence I had always been able to count on. Gone was the air of superiority I had carried before like a shield. I had just committed myself to do something for which there was no standard. The only example I had was what had happened to me in the dental office—on a weekend with no one else around, not even a hygienist. Here I was in the middle of the three-ring circus known as pre-op.

Mrs. Jones looked at me, concerned, as if to say, "Is there something new about the surgery? Something else I need to know? Should I be worried?" Like any other patient, she was highly attuned to the words and actions of her doctor, reading me for any clue about her status. Her daughters, too, stared at me, waiting for me to say something important, but I couldn't summon the courage. I felt as if I were about to drive my car off the highway and into the wilderness. Where would it lead? How was I going to introduce this subject? Would they think I was crazy and call off the surgery? I noticed the red emergency button on the wall of the room. It was for summoning nurses when urgent help was needed. Maybe one of the daughters, after hearing my offer to pray, would sidle over to the button and push it while keeping a wary eye on me.

Finally I could stand it no longer. I blurted out, "Can I pray with you?"

Mrs. Jones looked surprised, as if something had gone badly wrong since I last saw her. Then her face softened as she considered what I had said, and she responded, "Okay." I felt embarrassed but relieved. She was acting guarded and unsure about the offer. She seemed to be going along just to give me what I wanted. More than anything, she seemed confused. I imagine my offer was as unexpected as a pastor, priest, or rabbi asking if he or she could remove a mole during a counseling visit. I had no real choice but to press through it with some modicum of confidence.

Neurosurgeons don't mind touching people. We just prefer that they be washed with a sterile solution, covered with blue drape, and anesthetized first. Then we touch them only with a very sharp scalpel. Nevertheless, recalling how my dentist friend had put his hand on my shoulder, I carefully put my hand on Mrs. Jones's shoulder. As if by routine, her daughters moved in and bowed their heads. I froze. No words came. My mind was as blank as the whiteboard in my exam room.

I forced myself to start. "God, we thank you for Mrs. Jones . . ." It was an awkward beginning, small, not nearly what I had been hoping for. It reminded me of those tentative prayers given at Thanksgiving by children.

I paused. Then, I thought of whom we were talking to and not where we were. Out of nowhere, I felt a wind at my back, pushing me on. Without any forethought, the prayer began to flow like a river cascading downhill.

"God, you've been with Mrs. Jones since she was a baby. You know all about her vessels, and I know that you can help me fix them. Please give me wisdom and skill. I ask for success in this surgery, in the name of Jesus, Amen."

I looked up, not knowing what to expect. Mrs. Jones was crying and smiling peacefully. So were her two daughters. I was embarrassed and amazed. The prayer had been so brief that I couldn't believe it had produced such a dramatic and heartfelt response. I had closed my eyes seconds ago among three apparently skeptical people. When I opened my eyes, they had become puddles of emotion. My scientific side marveled.

I also felt a little flustered. I had not thought through the possible responses and certainly had not anticipated tears. What did it mean? I had no idea how to respond to their emotional display. Snapping back to my aloof professional manner, I decided to do what any emotionally vulnerable doctor would do: leave it for the nurse to deal with.

I patted Mrs. Jones's hand and turned away quickly. Sure enough, just as I was pulling aside the curtain, the nurse came back. *Right on time*, I thought. She surveyed the scene and handed them a box of tissues as I ducked out, hit the automatic door open button, and exited pre-op thinking, *Wow! What was that?* My heart was still pounding, but the peace and comfort that had brought Mrs. Jones to tears had also touched me. It wasn't the smoothest or even the most empathetic beginning, but I had done it. I had prayed with a patient. The world continued to spin. There were no shifts in the time-space continuum. I looked behind me in the hallway, but there was no squad of medical-industry police ready to grab me by my arms and hoist me onto an elevator, making sure I would never be seen practicing medicine again.

Rather, something wonderful had happened. Peace had overshadowed fear and created a different dynamic. It wasn't a dynamic that made sense to me yet or that I could describe, but something was different—and better.

Mrs. Jones's surgery went well. I treated the aneurysm

and noticed that I had unusual joy while performing the procedure—not something I had normally experienced during surgery. Certainly I always felt relief and happiness when a difficult case was over. The techs, doctors, and nurses are able to enjoy a certain banter involving cynical or gallows humor, and there might be light conversation about the ball game or something in the news. But once a neuro-endovascular procedure starts, there isn't a relaxed moment for me, because at any point something could go wrong and cause a stroke. That day, however, I felt lighthearted, free to perform well without fear hanging over me.

After the procedure was complete and Mrs. Jones woke up, I went into the waiting room. As is my custom, I called the family out into the hall to speak to them privately. The faces of the two young women were taut with concern and expectation.

"I'm happy to report that things went well," I said. They sighed audibly and smiles lit up their previously anxious faces.

I explained that their mother would be released the following day and gave them some post-op instructions so they would be aware of what she should do for the next couple of days. Then I asked them if they had any other questions.

They looked at each other, shared a moment of silent consultation, and the older one turned back to me.

"We wanted to tell you," she said, "that the prayer you said for our mother meant a lot to her—and to all of us. It really gave us all peace."

Now it was my turn to smile.

"I'm very glad," I said, trying to look appreciative and professional at the same time.

"We wanted to thank you for doing that," she said. The other nodded affirmatively.

Looking awkward, she continued, "Can we . . . hug you?" Her sister agreed and nodded.

"That would be fine," I said, and I hugged them individually. They were reaching in their purses for Kleenex as I walked down the hall toward the recovery room.

In their appreciation, I felt encouraged that I had done the right thing. I had another surgery that day, and I prayed with that patient as well. He was equally thankful. When I finally got home and had a chance to reflect on what I had done, I realized I had communicated something important and unusual to the patients. I was saying, in essence, "You may be looking to me for your outcome because of my skills, my confidence, and hopefully a glowing recommendation from other doctors, but I am willing to admit before you and your family that I am not God. I am good at what I do, but ultimately I cannot control the outcome of your surgery. Whether we like to admit it or not and no matter how simple or complex the case, my skills are not enough. We need God's help, and I am not ashamed to ask for it."

It required humility and honesty—and it felt great.

I also realized I had brought another dimension of the human experience into that room: the spiritual. When people have a spiritual experience, at best they feel that God is with them. At the least, prayer provides a catharsis for fear, which makes room for peace and hope during difficult times.

• • •

From that day forward I have offered to pray for nearly every patient before surgery. It has clearly blessed many people as they dealt with the illness and loss of control.

I began to actually enjoy surgery more than I had previously. Trying to control outcomes and therefore what people thought of me had taken the joy from my practice of medicine and from my life. Throughout my training I had used performance, perfectionism, and fear of failure to hone my technical skills. Adrenaline had been a necessary and welcome part of the job; I lived for the rush and the drama of a difficult procedure. I loved believing that my own intelligence and skill had snatched someone from the jaws of death. But when I took all the credit, I also took on all the pressure: constant stress, lack of sleep, the need to be absolutely perfect, and an overarching dread of failure or lawsuit. Of course, no one is absolutely perfect. Although I do have intelligence and skill, I believe I have been given them by God—which means I would not have them without him. When I began giving God the credit and responsibility for the outcome of my work, I realized that I could not remember a time when I had enjoyed the cases so much. By openly acknowledging that I was not God but that I worked for him and with him, I was able to stop carrying the entire burden on my shoulders.

A little while after I began praying with patients before surgery, it struck me that we were doing a lot of asking but not a lot of thanking God for the results. So I began praying with patients after surgery as well. When they awoke from anesthesia, I would lean over and whisper a prayer in their ear, thanking God for answering our pre-operative prayer and asking him to continue to guide and heal. If there was a problem, I would pray with them for the resolution.

When I first see patients in the office, I generally ask two questions related to "spiritual history": "In what faith or religion were you raised?" and "Are you practicing now?" This gives me some spiritual background on each patient and helps me not to offend anyone. As a surgeon, I want all my patients to know and feel that I personally care about their complete welfare, not just the part of their health for which they are seeing me. I want them to enjoy the best physical, emotional, and spiritual health possible, according to their own definitions. And I want to encourage them wherever they are on their spiritual journeys with their own faith, not to push my faith on them. It is not my job to insist that they address spiritual issues any more than I insist that they exercise, which is also good for health.

I generally offer to pray with everyone before surgery. I offer to pray with many patients I see in the office, as well, although I have no formula and do not offer to pray with every patient. If I don't think it will be a blessing, I don't offer. Then, if I detect any hesitation when I inquire about their emotional and spiritual health, I make sure they know that I did not mean to make them uncomfortable and that my desire is for their total health. Then I move right along to other topics. It is not right or productive to force them in any particular direction. My job, as I see it, is to give them the opportunity to make good choices in all areas pertaining to their health. I make it safe to accept or reject the offer.

Nothing had changed about how I performed surgery. I still strove to be the best and took great satisfaction in complex cases that required high-level skills and performance. Nevertheless, the way I related to patients had changed forever—with consequences I could never have expected.

CHAPTER 3

INTRODUCING
SPIRITUAL CARE

ONE DAY THE RECEPTIONIST at my practice came back to my office looking puzzled and a bit uncertain.

"There's a woman here to see you," she said. "She doesn't have an appointment, but she says you operated on her a year ago."

This was unusual—most people don't just drop in on their neurosurgeon—but I had a few moments to spare in my schedule.

"Send her back," I replied, wondering who this woman might be and what was so urgent that would make her come by unannounced.

Moments later a former patient entered my office.

I immediately recognized the confident woman and remembered her case. Her name was Joan. She was petite with dark hair and looked much younger than her advanced years. She had taken good care of herself, and she had the appearance of someone in control and perfectly put together. She had been referred to me because a dangerous aneurysm had been discovered in her brain. Instead of being a single round ball, the aneurysm was multilobed with a wide neck. This type is harder and riskier to repair, and you never know if you can do the surgery without blocking the main blood vessel. We had spent a lot of time going over the pros and cons of doing the procedure, in light of her age and ability to endure and recover from it. With nearly eighty-year-old vessels, she could easily have had a stroke if devices were maneuvered through them.

The aneurysm looked ugly, as though it could bleed at any time, and I did feel she should have it fixed. But given her age, I could not suggest one course of action more strongly than another. I could only provide the statistics and let her decide. She had brought her family in to help her make the decision. After deliberating, they decided to go forward with surgery. I prayed with her before and after the procedure. At that time, she let me know rather firmly that she didn't believe in God but that she did not mind if I prayed for her.

The surgery went well. Joan's follow-up examination had indicated no lingering complications. There was no reason to see me again. Yet there she stood in my office, one year later, looking a little out of place but self-possessed, as I remembered her. Her words were unexpected.

"I came here without any makeup and without an appointment because I just needed to see you," she said. I had no idea what to make of her urgency, so I did what most smart doctors do: I leaned back against my desk, put my head to one side, and listened.

"At my last appointment after the surgery, I asked you a question," she continued. "I asked why most educated people don't believe in God, and you said you thought it was because they were arrogant."

I nodded and smiled. That did not sound like something I would have said, although I did remember her asking the provocative question. Whatever I had said, this was her interpretation of it.

"I can't get what you said out of my head," she exclaimed, glaring at me with irritation. I didn't quite know how to respond, so I decided to take a safe path by eliciting some general information.

"Tell me how things are going in your life," I asked.

"Not very well," she sighed. "My husband had a stroke recently. It's been causing us trouble. He's not recovering like we hoped he would. Life seems to have taken a turn for the worse for both of us. We don't know where to find answers."

She paused.

"I needed to talk to someone about faith," she said, in a tone of embarrassment.

The irony of this conversation did not escape me. I had not seen her for a year and didn't expect to ever see her again. Yet when Joan needed someone to turn to in her time of deepest need, she chose to confide in me—her neurosurgeon. Without her makeup, no less.

"Tell me about your faith," I said, giving her an open door to talk about her concerns.

"I don't think I can believe in the Bible," she replied, charging right into the crux of her dilemma. "I don't see how I can believe in Jesus. So many highly educated and intelligent people think it's simply a myth."

Realizing that this conversation would probably need to go beyond the five minutes I had to spare, I knew I had to postpone it while I took care of a patient who actually had an appointment.

"Joan, I need to meet with another patient. That should take about thirty minutes, and then I have a break for lunch," I said. "In the meantime, take this pad of paper into the waiting room and write down all the reasons you don't believe in God. Write down anything standing between you and God: people who have hurt you, people who were supposed to represent God and did it poorly, things you prayed about but didn't get, painful experiences, and anything you feel guilty about."

Something else occurred to me. Joan's resistance to faith might stem from valuing too highly the opinions of educated people, many of whom considered faith to be a fairy tale, something only the unsophisticated would believe. Based on our previous conversation, I knew she had such people in her family.

"I want you to do one more thing too," I added. "Ask yourself whether, if the story of Jesus were true, you would want to believe it. You may find many reasons why, even if it is true, you wouldn't want to believe it. You may not want to be 'one of those people.' You may not want to lose the respect of people you love. Maybe you don't want to be religiously or politically stereotyped. Maybe you think that to believe God came to earth would be to deny your intellect. Whether it's true or not may not be the issue. You may not want to believe it."

Startled, Joan looked at me as if this question had never occurred to her. It was as if I had switched on a light in a room she had never seen in her own house. I also sensed fear that if she came to believe, she might be the only one in her marriage, family, or social circle who had faith. She was wisely counting the cost, and it appeared steep. She took the paper and walked out. Part of me wondered if I would ever see her again.

When I was finished with my other patient, I walked out to the waiting room. Joan was sitting there with the piece of paper covered in her handwriting. She handed it to me. At the top of the page it read, somewhat momentously, "My List." We walked back to my office and I began to read. First on her list of objections were her parents, particularly her mother, who had been unkind to her throughout her childhood. Joan saw hypocrisy in the church they attended, where many people, including her parents, kept up appearances while acting badly at home. When she was fourteen, Joan decided her parents' view of God couldn't be correct and went on a spiritual journey to find God, attending several churches. She then found a boy she liked who didn't go to church, and she stopped searching for God. She felt that she had made a reasonable effort and had come up empty. Besides, this boy seemed like a better deal.

The boy Joan met would become her husband. She was only fifteen when they began a physical relationship. She felt justified rebelling against her parents' rules and morals because of her failure to find God and because of her parents' hypocrisy. Even so, deep down she felt ashamed and guilty, which pushed her further from God. That was sixty-five years ago. She had never again searched for God, until now. She had noted at least one affair on the list, with her family doctor, who had told her sex would help her depression. It worked for a while, until he shot himself.

For some reason, I felt free to speak openly with Joan. After all, this time she had come to me not as her physician but as a spiritual counselor.

"Did you feel guilty?" I asked.

She had obviously been thinking about what started her on this godless journey and answered quickly, "Oh, it was terrible. I would see my mother in the kitchen and I could have just died, I felt so guilty."

"The reason we feel guilty is usually because we are guilty," I said, not knowing how she would respond. Perhaps she would storm out of my office. I continued, "We are guilty of going against what we know is right, even if we justify it because of what others do or say. God calls it sin. The good news is that there is a cure for guilt and sin. It is confession and forgiveness."

She shook her head rather violently.

"I won't do that," she said. "I don't see sin that way."

Joan's resistance was vehement. I have learned from doing surgery that when you meet resistance, you can't keep pushing harder. Instead, you try to understand what is blocking your way. When operating in the brain, pushing harder can burst a blood vessel and kill the patient. Regarding spiritual matters, also, I believe that pushing when you meet resistance causes more harm than good.

I scaled back our conversation. Looking at her, I thought about how in control she wanted to be. Many people would have envied her had they seen her in public or met her at a social function. She had an elegant demeanor and exuded a quiet inner confidence. Nobody could see the hidden turmoil raging inside.

"I think the reason you're here," I responded after a quiet moment, "is that you've been able to control everything in your life up to now. You've made things work. You have been able to keep God out of your life because your health has been good and your marriage has been good. Even your aneurysm treatment went perfectly. Everything has been working for you. But that facade is falling apart. Now that your husband is debilitated, you are asking whether there could be anything more to life. I imagine you came to me because you are asking yourself when you last saw someone with hope."

She agreed with me in her silence. After a few moments she responded.

"I know I haven't lived a perfect life," she said. This was

a familiar phrase to me. In essence sin is simply missing the mark or not being perfect. People prefer to think of it as an honest mistake, instead of a willing choice. They often cannot tolerate the word *sin* because it implies that someone is judging their actions. Instead, they use softer, more palatable euphemisms, as Joan was doing.

"To get rid of the guilty feelings, I bet you shut down whatever faith you had," I continued. "You stopped looking for God. You didn't want it to be true."

I seemed to have told the story of her life, and she seemed to be listening.

"So, what do I do?" she finally inquired.

My reply was heartfelt: "I would love to help you with your sin, but I can't, because I have my own. What you need is someone who has no sin, someone who lived a perfect life. Then he would be able to pay for your sin because he has none of his own. That is why Jesus came to earth, lived a perfect life, and died—to get rid of whatever sins and guilt are blocking you from being in relationship with God. He actually wants to take your guilt from you and leave you free from shame. Guilt comes naturally when we sin, and you can try to pay for sin yourself by feeling shame, or you can let Jesus pay for it and be forgiven. I believe that he really wants to forgive you, but it requires confession."

She thought a moment, looking doubtful, but then seemed to conclude that she wasn't going to leave without trying something. After all, desperation had driven her to my office in the first place.

"Do I have to?" she asked.

"No, not at all," I replied, "but I don't know any other way to get rid of guilt. I can help you find excuses for what you did to try to make you feel better, but I can't forgive you. The fact is you have already spent years justifying what you did—including trying to convince yourself that there is no God—and claiming that you are not guilty. But here you are, still feeling guilty."

"What about other religions?" she asked, and I was not about to push her into something she was not ready to do.

"You are welcome to investigate other religions," I said. "Take all the time you need. The questions I think you need to ask of each one are, 'How do I get forgiveness?' and 'How do I know I am forgiven?'"

"Okay," she said softly.

"Would you like Jesus to pay for your sins?" I asked.

"Yes," she said.

"Do you need more time to think about it?" I asked.

She shook her head and replied, "No."

"Do you want me to help you talk to God?" I asked.

"Yes," she said.

I began to pray on her behalf while Joan looked out my office window, deep in consideration.

"God, you know everything about Joan," I said. "You know the good and the bad. Only you have the power to take away our guilt and to forgive us. Joan would like to do that now."

"Joan, think about what I am saying, and if you agree with it, you say it. 'God, I have sinned.'"

After a moment she said, "God, I have sinned. I knew what I was doing was wrong, but I did it anyway."

She paused, contemplating carefully, and then said again, with conviction, "I knew what I was doing was wrong, but I did it anyway. Forgive my rebellion."

We continued, with me offering suggestions and Joan stating them in her own words: "Jesus, thank you for paying for my sins so I can be free of my guilt. Thank you for forgiving me like you promised. Amen."

She was still staring out the window. She did not look any different. She showed no sign of emotion. There was not even a hint of tears. She remained stiff, prim, unflappable. Still, I marveled at this intelligent woman who, decades earlier, had walked away from God for a boy who didn't want God. Disbelief had left her unfulfilled. Now she was searching for God again and was ready to give faith another chance.

"I feel a lightness," she finally said, "like I have a cloud inside me."

She stood there experiencing this euphoric, peaceful feeling, seeming to analyze and enjoy it at the same time.

"You are feeling some of the joy that God feels now that you two are talking again," I said with a smile. "Sin is God's least favorite subject. He must deal with it to remove your guilt and convince you that nothing is blocking the relationship between you. But he really wants to hear you speak to him about what matters to you. That's what prayer is."

"How do I . . . start?" she asked.

"I usually start with gratitude," I said. "It helps my mood

and stops me from focusing on negative things. Just tell him what you are thankful for."

She shifted in her seat. "Well, God, . . . thank you that I've been healthy most of my life. And my aneurysm surgery went well; I'm thankful for that."

"That's a great start," I said. "There is so much that we take for granted. What else? If I get stuck, I start with my eyes. There are a lot of people who cannot see."

"Yes, thank you, God, that I can see and hear and walk," she said.

"Don't forget your mind. Not everyone has a sharp mind at your age," I added.

She went on giving thanks for a few minutes, becoming more joyful as she realized all that she had been taking for granted.

"My granddaughter, the apple of my eye—I am thankful for her."

"You know," I said, "the way you think about your granddaughter is the way God thinks about you. He adores you."

"Really? I never thought of God like that."

"He would also love to hear about anything that concerns you, like your husband's illness," I said.

Joan then spoke to God with confidence about her concerns for her husband.

Finally, I said, "Any good relationship requires both talking and listening. I think you already know how to listen to God."

"I do?" She sat up straight, surprised.

"Why else would you rush in to see your neurosurgeon

to talk about faith, with no appointment—and no makeup?" I smiled. "Who do you think gave you that idea?"

She raised her eyebrows. Indeed, this had not been like her.

I felt deeply thankful. I had witnessed something price-less. My day had taken an unexpected but wonderful turn. Joan stepped forward and hugged me somewhat formally. Then I walked her to the door. As difficult as she was to read, I could tell she was a different woman from the one who had barged into my office earlier. Her presence felt easier, fresh and new. The lines in her face were softer. I don't often get to see the results of my providential encounters with patients, but I had just watched a woman move toward the One who, out of his great love, could forgive any sin and free her from the guilt and shame she carried. I cannot think of a better way to use my lunch hour than to help someone talk to God—because once the two of them are talking, the pos-sibilities for healing go way beyond me.[1]

• • •

Once I began praying with patients, it didn't take long to realize that I would not actually get to observe a change or difference in the lives of most of them because our inter-actions were necessarily brief. There was no reasonable way to follow up with them even for medical reasons. I rarely got a bird's-eye view of their faith journeys—I was privy to only a small snapshot along the way that took place during extraordinary circumstances. All I could do was offer some semblance of peace during a time of crisis and perform the procedure to the best of my ability; most went their own way to recover. No one could blame them for wanting to stay away from hospitals after what they had been through. If they were impacted by our interactions, I had no way to know unless they sent me a card or note in the months after surgery. Enough people thanked me that I felt encouraged to keep going, but I assumed that I was making little difference in the day-to-day lives of most people. I rested in the knowledge that I had given them all I could to make their lives better, even if some might find it odd that their doctor would pray.

Occasionally, patients did come back to the hospital to share their stories. One kind woman in her sixties, Gloria, came by my office to review a follow-up scan. I had last seen her six months earlier and had counseled her about a benign tangle of extraneous vessels in the back of her head, as well as some small aneurysms we were following with scans. Her follow-up scan showed no change in the aneurysms, and we decided not to pursue surgery.

"Do you remember the friend who came with me last time?" Gloria asked after we had finished talking about the facts of her case.

"Sort of, but not exactly," I admitted.

"I brought my friend Gail with me for support, remember? You said a prayer for me at the end of the visit."

"I'm sure I did," I said, without having any specific recollection.

"Well, after you prayed for me, we left your office, went outside into the hallway, and just held each other and wept. We couldn't figure out why we were crying. This was highly unusual for both of us. We just felt this need to cry after leaving your office."

I was intrigued by this. I would not have imagined that kind of response to a simple prayer for her health.

"About a week later," Gloria continued, "my friend told me she wanted to have a relationship with God and asked for my help. I took her to church, where Gail went to talk to the pastor and make peace with God."

"That's wonderful," I said.

"A few weeks later," Gloria continued, "Gail found out she had cancer. A month later she died. Within three months of that appointment with you, I was at her funeral."

I was stunned. I didn't even know what to say. She spoke instead.

"I just wanted to thank you, Dr. Levy, for not being afraid to bring up the option of prayer," she concluded. "It made a world of difference in my friend's life."

She gave me a quick hug as we walked out of my office. I went through the rest of my day with a profound feeling that even the smallest of decisions can have huge impact on the lives of people I interact with daily, or on the people they bring with them whom I don't even notice. It often appeared to me that nothing significant happens as a result of my prayers, but I have learned that there is much that I don't get to see.

• • •

By this time nearly all the patients I prayed with were wel-coming and appreciative. They seemed pleasantly surprised to discover a neurosurgeon addressing physical, emotional, and spiritual needs while in the midst of what is often a ster-ile, impersonal environment. My patients seemed genuinely caught off guard when I would make them partners in asking for God's help in their cases. There was something "undoctorly" and humble about relating to them as human beings.

Even laying a hand on patients' shoulders or holding their hands felt strange at first, as though I were violating their personal space. In an environment where touch tends to be cold, mechanical, and sterile, I was touching them out of kindness. This touch was professional yet had a purpose that couldn't be listed as an item to be checked off on a patient's chart. It was not the routine touch of someone taking a pulse or fitting a medical band around a wrist, the kind that is purely clinical and that can make any patient feel like a petri dish specimen. It was a touch that, when offered properly and appropriately, conveyed concern, connected two lives, and spoke to the soul. Touching a shoulder or holding hands with a patient or family member, when welcome and always within the bounds of medical decorum, became a leveling and personal experience that said, "We are all human and we're in this together, each doing our part."

Naturally, some people probably agree to pray with me only because I am about to meddle in their brains. I am always keenly aware of the patients' vulnerability while they are lying on gurneys wearing only hospital gowns, with IVs dangling from their arms, waiting to be wheeled away so someone could insert a tube up half the length of their bodies and operate on the inside of their skulls. For the patient, this is not your typical day. So the obvious answer when a surgeon approaches you in pre-op and asks if he can pray with you is probably going to be, "Okay." I have had some of those responses. A patient will sometimes look at me askance or with resignation and say, "Whatever you want, Doc. Whatever's good for you." Yet most people seem visibly comforted, even those who claim not to believe in God. I have seen many tears and often feel the atmosphere of the room change from tension to peaceful anticipation.

At some point I even began to rely on this atmospheric shift and look forward to calming fear with prayer. In that moment of petition we could forget we were in a busy pre-op or exam room. We could put ourselves, doctor and patient together, into the hands of God. These experiences became as much a part of my workday as the surgical procedures themselves. I came to enjoy prayer as much as any other part of my routine, because it invited a peace and perspective that helped not only the patient and the family but also me. The best we could do in purely medical terms was to give patients a sedative to reduce their fear chemically. But to also address that fear on a spiritual and emotional level was natural, beautiful, and real. It offered what science lacked—medicine for the soul.

I was now being authentic about who I was and what I

believed, so I was caring for my own soul too. I have always been a perfectionist, as you would want your neurosurgeon to be, and I had also experienced the downside of that approach to the world. Now I was a more relaxed neurosurgeon, a happier perfectionist. I felt mentally and physically better prepared to handle the unexpected challenges that surface during surgery on the blood vessels of the brain. I was certainly better able to handle angry or out-of-control family members. I even felt that providing spiritual care was actually making me a better doctor.

Sometimes encouragement in my new course of action came inconveniently. One woman, Rosa, a retiree, had an aneurysm and persistent headaches. I treated the aneurysm, but her headaches persisted. This was a common result and simply meant that the two problems were unrelated. Aneurysms can be indicated by severe headaches, but most people with headaches do not have aneurysms. I saw Rosa several times and made repeated scans to check that the treatment had worked. She was convinced that the headaches should have stopped if the procedure had been successful. I tried to explain that this was not always the case and that the aneurysm had been repaired correctly. There was nothing more I could do for her. But she couldn't understand why she was still having headaches.

Finally, partly out of exasperation, I offered to pray for her headaches just as I had prayed for her before and after surgery. Rosa agreed. I put my hand gently on her head and asked God to take away her headaches. When the short prayer was done, she said, "Thank you, Doctor. I feel better." And then she walked out the door.

I was not expecting to see her again. About six months later I was surprised when I saw her name on my schedule. I asked my receptionist why she'd been given an appointment—I had nothing to offer. She said Rosa had insisted on seeing me. I had been looking for time to add yet another patient into my packed schedule, yet there Rosa was in my exam room.

Pausing at the door to the exam room, I put a smile on my face and decided that I would treat her with respect even though I was already behind schedule and knew that another consultation was a waste of time. I walked into the room to find her surrounded by her loved ones—children, grand-children, and other family friends. Rosa was smiling and happy to see me.

"What can I do for you today?" I asked, sitting on my rolling stool and smiling pleasantly as if I had all the time in the world.

"I'm having headaches again," she said.

I gritted my teeth, trying to be kind.

"As I told you before, there is nothing more I can do for you," I said. "We have looked at the angiograms together. Your aneurysm was repaired and is not causing your head-aches. There's nothing more I can do."

Then, as a consolation, I added, "But if you want, I'd be glad to pray for you again."

She looked at me as though I were the one who didn't understand.

"But that's why I'm here, Doctor," she said. "I don't want pills or another surgery. When you prayed for me last time, my headaches went away. A few weeks ago they came back, so I'm here to have you pray for me again."

She smiled and settled in, ready to receive. Feeling contrite and a bit relieved, I walked over, put my hand on her head, and prayed for her headaches to go away. After I said "Amen," she smiled and said, "Thank you," as if to say, "Was that too much to ask?" She had been given just the prescription she wanted. Her family members smiled, shook my hand, and thanked me profusely as they left. I never saw Rosa again.

• • •

Tears became common during and after my meetings with patients, and I quickly learned not to be flustered or alarmed by emotion. I began to see tears as an indicator of something positive, an honest reaction to fear or to feeling cared for. Patients felt safe to display feelings in my office that they could not display at home or with friends. I became comfortable with tears and simply handed out tissues. Many times a patient would leave my office dabbing his or her eyes after we had consulted and prayed together.

I only realized how common this emotional response had become when I walked into the exam room one day and introduced myself to Darla, a thin, fit, blonde woman in her late forties. This was our initial consultation for an aneurysm on the carotid artery in her neck that needed attention.

I extended my hand and introduced myself.

"You're not going to make me cry, are you?" she asked immediately.

I was taken aback. Nobody had ever said that to me. I must have worn my puzzlement on my face.

"Because I don't have my waterproof mascara on," she said, "and I need to go back to work after this appointment."

I was so caught off guard that I didn't even ask why she thought I would make her cry, but I reassured her I would not. We proceeded to talk about the facts of her case. Reflecting on it later, I thought she may have seen other patients reenter the waiting room crying and wondered exactly what was in store for her.

As common as the good responses are, not all patients are eager to have God addressed or acknowledged during their visits to the doctor. Some are annoyed, some resistant, and some downright hostile. I have had to learn how to handle those types of people with grace as well.

CHAPTER 4

SKEPTICS

ALTHOUGH MOST OF MY PATIENTS appreciate spiritual care, some want nothing to do with it. Diane, a forty-three-year-old businesswoman, came to see me with a host of physical problems. Aside from the irregularity in her brain, she had diabetes, kidney trouble, skin problems, depression, and a number of other afflictions. It was going to take a lot of doctors and medical attention to make her well. She mentioned during our appointment that she had been treated poorly by people in her past. It was clear to me that she saw herself as a victim, and it was easy to feel sorry for her. I recommended she see a professional counselor, and at the end of that appointment I offered to pray with her. She agreed.

The next time I saw her, a year had gone by. She came in for a checkup. Her repeat scan showed no progression of her small aneurysm. She told me she had started going to counseling, was getting a lot stronger physically, and was off antidepressants. I celebrated the good news with her. Just before the appointment ended, I said, "I would be glad to say a prayer for you."

"No," Diane said, turning suddenly cold. "I'm learning to be more assertive about what I want and don't want. And I don't want prayer."

I smiled and told her that was okay with me and that I appreciated her letting me know her wishes. I walked her to the waiting room, put my hand on her shoulder, and smiled.

"You have come a long way," I said. She smiled and thanked me. She was enjoying her assertiveness, and I took no offense.

Another couple had a New Age belief system that was unclear to me. They were young, wealthy, and professional. The husband had a type of neurological disease that had no medical solution. Surgery would not help him. As the appointment came to a close and they were about to leave, I offered, "I would be glad to pray with you."

"No. We have our own beliefs," replied the woman sharply. The husband said nothing but looked soberly down at the floor. This couple's response fit an interesting pattern: it is almost always the healthy partner who steps in and says "no thanks" to prayer. The person with the brain problem almost always welcomes prayer, or at least tolerates it.

One of the saddest episodes to take place in my exam room involved a devoutly atheistic family. Sally, the elderly mother of the family, had denied the existence of God her entire life and raised her children to believe that God was a myth for weak-minded people. Now Sally had a degenerative brain disease that neither medicine nor surgery could correct. She was fragile and clearly approaching the end of her life. As our consultation concluded, I offered to pray for her. Sally's adult son and daughter virtually launched themselves between us.

"No, no, we don't believe that," the son exclaimed. They planted themselves next to their mother like bodyguards protecting her from imminent danger. But I could see that their mother was deeply torn. Sally had not turned down my offer. Her eyes pleaded with me in some unspoken way. A great sadness came over me.

"I'm asking her," I said calmly, trying to avoid an incident with her son. All three of us looked at their mother, but she wouldn't say anything.

"She doesn't believe that," the son repeated, as though he were trying to convince his mother of her own beliefs. The daughter chimed in, as if to warn me off: "She doesn't believe that."

Sally sat there, uncertain, saying nothing. She seemed unbearably sad and clearly desired the hope she had detected in my offer. The four of us held our tense silence. Briefly, I considered asking Sally's children to leave the room, but that would have been too confrontational. Finally, there was nothing more to do or say.

"Okay, then let's go out to the front desk," I said. The old woman looked numb. Her children helped her get up and collect her things. I led them silently out of the room, but I was left with a hollow, chilled feeling. She had convinced her children that God did not exist. Now, probably in her final days, they were there to return the favor and make sure she did not stray from the family belief—the belief that there was nothing and no one outside our medical system to help her.

• • •

On one occasion, it was prayer that alerted a patient to the seriousness of the operation he was about to undergo, even though this was not my intention.

Daniel was a British man in his sixties who wore a handle-bar mustache and was unfailingly jolly. Every other comment of his was a lighthearted joke. He didn't seem to take life too seriously, and that included his brain ailment and his medical treatment. He was also a longtime smoker. Every time I saw him, his wife, Nellie, was with him. They seemed close and very much in love after many years of marriage.

Daniel had a basilar tip aneurysm, one of the more difficult kinds of aneurysms to treat. It was bell shaped, with a wide neck. The basilar artery travels in front of the brain stem and divides, forming a T at the very top. A basilar tip aneurysm forms when the wall of the vessel is weak, and the blood doesn't stop at the T but pushes out the opposite wall, creating a bubble on top.

To repair a brain aneurysm through the blood vessels (the endovascular route), we fill it with soft platinum coils, which reinforce it and prevent it from growing, like filling a pothole with asphalt. The coils go into the catheter straight and then assume a spherical shape once inserted into the vessel. These ingenious little devices come in different sizes, from 1.5 to 24 millimeters in globelike configurations. It is much easier to repair a narrow-necked aneurysm, which has a wide bottom and narrow neck, resembling a balloon, because the neck can hold the platinum coils inside. A bell-shaped, wide-necked aneurysm has nothing to keep the coils from spilling out and blocking the native vessels and therefore the blood flow to the brain. For Daniel's aneurysm, I would need to use a stent and possibly other devices to re-create the wall of the vessel before inserting platinum coils, which would act as blocking agents. Each additional device would mean additional risk to the procedure.

I explained the risks to Daniel and Nellie in detail. He seemed to shrug them off. I thought perhaps this was how he handled stress. The medical-consent form echoed what I said and made abundantly clear all the possible disasters that could befall him, including death. This was a high-risk procedure; the chances of having a stroke, being paralyzed, or even dying as a result were well above normal. He casually signed the form, appearing to put the risks immediately out of mind.

While he was lying on the gurney awaiting surgery, I asked, as I normally do, if I could pray for him. Daniel's ever-present smile suddenly disappeared, and his wife looked at me with concern. It seemed as if they were asking themselves, Did we hear this guy right? Are we in a hospital? Did the neurosurgeon just ask if we wanted to pray?

"Okay," Daniel said after an awkward hesitation. So I said a brief prayer. When I opened my eyes, I could tell that, like many others, they had kept their eyes open the whole time. Daniel looked like a deer in headlights. His mood had changed completely: he was stunned and quiet, and he even looked pale. The joking and easy conversation stopped. I wondered about his change in disposition as I told Nellie I would see her in the waiting room after surgery.

Daniel's procedure proved to be extremely difficult. The aneurysm was located as expected at the T-shaped intersection in his brain, where a vessel branches off into two opposite directions. This is a common place to find an aneurysm, but this case was not common.

In Daniel's case, just getting to the T-shaped junction with the catheter was arduous. His vessels were horribly diseased from all the years of smoking. The vertebral artery, the vessel I was trying to use as our passageway into his brain, had a kink and stenosis—a narrowing within. Just getting past these took two hours as I gingerly maneuvered the catheter through the calcified and fragile vessel.

Even in a healthy person with wide-open arteries and veins, getting to the diseased area in the brain is often more difficult than, say, in the heart or other parts of the body. This is because of the tight corners to get around as the arteries enter the skull. The carotid or vertebral arteries, which begin in the chest, travel through the neck and become the brain vessels, taking multiple hairpin turns as they enter the skull. This tortuosity of the vessels, as well as the fact that the curves cannot be straightened because of the bone structure, means that the devices you would use in heart surgery will not work in brain surgery. The stents, wires, and catheters have to be much softer and more flexible. It is delicate and tricky territory no matter how healthy the patient. With Daniel it was much more difficult.

I found I couldn't even enter Daniel's vertebral artery with the guide catheter because the vessel was so hardened with plaque. The artery was much narrower than normal and had hard little bumps all around the inside, like the surface of a gravel road. This put us at a major disadvantage because without a catheter in the artery we could not see clearly what we were doing. Usually, I inject dye through the guide catheter directly into the artery so my team can snap a movielike series of X-ray pictures to see where the instruments are positioned in relation to the aneurysm, and so on. Because the guide catheter could not be brought into the entrance of the vertebral artery, which was only inches away from the heart, the dye was diluted and didn't give us good quality pictures. Not only that but, as is common, the vessels I was working on had moved because of the introduction of my instruments. The aneurysm was not even in the same place it had been, so getting a new visual was even more important. Frustratingly, I just couldn't get the dye up to where I needed it.

The human body has two vertebral arteries that supply the brain stem and upper spine with blood. I was now blocking one with the catheter; the other was picking up the slack, but it was very small and could do that for only a limited time. I did not know how long; I just knew that the sooner we pulled out of his vertebral artery, the sooner his brain stem would have its full supply of oxygenated blood. Daniel's case was taking much longer than we had hoped. I wanted to move quickly, but the disease in the vessels was causing delays at every turn.

I felt around the insides of the vessels with the wires, sliding them along blindly using feel, experience, and my imagination to "see" the shape of the vessel since the road-map scan we had made was no longer accurate. My goal was to re-create the aneurysm neck with stents so I could then block off the weakened part of the wall with platinum micro-coils. These tiny coils feel very soft; they are used to fill space and act as a resistor so blood no longer flows there. They have a helical shape and want to form a ball. The body eventually solidifies around the ball. This is the common medical way of patching a weak point in a vessel wall.

Normally you check the position of the aneurysm in relation to the stent before deploying the stent. In this case we couldn't, because we couldn't get a decent picture. If I did not properly place the stent, I ran the risk that the coils would slip out of the aneurysm and block the vessel itself, causing a major stroke.

I placed the stent across the neck of the aneurysm, inserted the amount of coil I believed was needed to fix the aneurysm, and then waited. Daniel's vitals remained normal. We took a final-run angiogram to see if the aneurysm was repaired and all the vessels in his head were filling with blood. We noticed that the vertebral artery in the neck looked a little bit rough, as if the walls had been slightly damaged during the procedure; usually this type of damage would heal on blood thinners, which Daniel had been taking. His vessels were in such bad shape to begin with and had endured so much during the surgery that the damage seemed par for the course. The angiogram showed us that all the sizable vessels in the brain had good blood flow. There was nothing more for us to do. I removed the wires and catheters and sealed the puncture site in the femoral artery with a clip device.

My team and I breathed a collective sigh when the lengthy procedure was over, but we never feel real relief until a patient wakes up and is able to talk and move his or her fingers and toes. Only then do we know how the procedure has gone. There is still much we do not understand about the brain— the fact that the angiography and scans look good doesn't guarantee that the patient will wake up neurologically normal. Until that happens, we feel suspended in time.

I went to get a drink of water, then began reviewing the angiography images and writing in the chart while waiting for Daniel to wake up from the anesthesia. Most patients wake up in fifteen minutes or so. If they are obese, which Daniel was not, it might take longer to wake up because the drugs get stored in the fat and are processed out over a longer time. At a certain point, Daniel's anesthesiologist said that by now the drugs should be out of his system—and still he was not waking up. Had something happened during his surgery that I was not aware of? To my relief, the CT scan showed no hemorrhage.

After an hour and a half, he fluttered his eyes. A little while later, when most patients are able to carry on a conversation, Daniel could hardly speak. When he tried, his words were slurred, and he couldn't move one side of his body. It looked as if he'd had an embolic stroke. An MRI scan confirmed a small stroke, but not just any stroke—it was in the brain stem.

There are two kinds of strokes. An embolic (or ischemic) stroke is caused by a piece of plaque from the arterial wall or a blood clot that lodges in an artery and stops the blood flow, depriving brain cells of critically needed oxygen. Bleeding (hemorrhagic) strokes occur when an aneurysm or vessel ruptures and blood goes into the brain. We were trying to prevent a bleeding stroke by fixing Daniel's aneurysm. In the process, he had an embolic stroke instead.

Relative to other parts of the brain, the brain stem has important functions packed in a very small area. Nerve fibers taking the commands and information from the surface of the brain come together like a funnel as they travel through the brain stem on their way to the spinal cord. The brain stem is the center of consciousness, involuntary and essential functions such as breathing, and much more. People can stay alive without their frontal lobes, but not without their brain stems. A small stroke that might not be noticed in the forebrain can cause hemiparesis (weakness on one side of the body) or worse if it occurs in the brain stem.

I was fairly certain that a piece of cholesterol plaque must have come loose from Daniel's vertebral artery and lodged in a small artery feeding the brain stem. Too small for us to see on an angiogram but large enough to cause damage, the piece of cholesterol blocked blood from reaching that small part of the brain stem. Over the next few hours it became apparent that Daniel was not the same person he had been when he went in for surgery, and his prognosis became uncertain: He might get worse. He might get better. He might remain paralyzed. He might not regain function or speech. He had been pretreated with blood thinners before the surgery, and his blood thinners, which now were the only treatment available for his stroke, were continued after the surgery. There was nothing more I could do for him medically or surgically.

Once we had a handle on what had likely happened, I went to talk to Nellie and escorted her out of the waiting room and into a passageway.

"The surgery to repair the aneurysm appears to have been successful, but Daniel had a stroke during surgery," I said. "The procedure was very difficult because of his diseased vessels. I wish I could tell you what the final outcome will be, but I can't. It's very much up in the air right now. Many stroke victims recover significantly, and we are doing everything we can to treat Daniel's new situation."

Nellie took this in, then looked at me questioningly.

"Did you know he was going to have a stroke?" she asked.

"Pardon me?" I said, thinking I had misheard her.

"Did you know he was going to have a stroke? Is that why you prayed?" she asked again.

The question confounded me for a moment.

"No," I said, "I didn't know he was going to have a stroke. It's my habit to ask to pray with everyone before surgery."

"Because that really scared him—when you prayed," she said. "He didn't think it was serious before that."

I was surprised, but this explained his turning somber and quiet afterward.

"This was a very high-risk surgery, and I thought I had made that clear," I said. "But no, I didn't know he would have a stroke. I ask to pray with everyone."

Nellie seemed unsettled by the stroke but satisfied that I hadn't known beforehand that it would happen. I accompanied her back to the waiting room. Daniel was slow to recover, but over time he regained much of the function he had lost. They both came and saw me for a follow-up six months later. I had no idea how the experience had affected them long term, if it had at all. My hope, naturally, was not only that he continue to regain his physical function but that they were prompted into a fresh consideration of their spiritual beliefs. That remains between them and God.

• • •

Often the reluctant person is a family member, and in one case it was the highly educated grandfather of a very bright eight-year-old girl named Tina. Tina was in the gifted program at school, played the saxophone, and excelled in language arts and history. One day while playing her instrument, Tina discovered she could not breathe through her right nostril. Decongestants didn't work, so the family took her in to have her checked out. A scan showed a large vascular tumor sitting against the carotid artery and filling the entire right side of her face. It was even causing her cheek to bulge in one area.

Tina came to see me with her parents, Tammy and Richard, and her grandfather, Dr. Willard, who I soon learned was a retired medical doctor affiliated with Harvard University. He wanted the girl to go to Boston for treatment at one of the academic hospitals he was familiar with. I told him that I felt comfortable doing the procedure but that he was welcome to get a second opinion wherever he liked. Because of the risks involved, it was important that they have confidence in whoever was going to do the surgery.

At our consultation, I recommended embolization, which means blocking the blood supply to the tumor with a "glue" injected through the artery. Embolization would be dangerous in this case, because the tumor was getting blood from the ophthalmic artery and other arteries off the carotid. If the glue went into these arteries, it could cause blindness or stroke. The procedure would also take many hours and therefore require a significant amount of radiation. A second surgery, done by our excellent skull base surgery team, would require an incision under Tina's eye and down the side of her nose to open up the facial area and remove the tumor, which was invading the temporal lobe of the brain.

Although Tammy and Richard had confidence in me and wanted to have the surgery in San Diego, Dr. Willard wanted his granddaughter treated across the country, in Boston. Under somewhat awkward conditions, Tina's parents decided to move forward with my embolization procedure, followed a few days later by open surgery to remove the tumor. When they returned for the pre-operative visit, Dr. Willard was sitting with the rest of the family. I could tell that he had not warmed up to the idea of my treating Tina, and I felt he was watching me for any slipup that would signal a lack of professionalism. Once again I explained the risks to them. Then I turned to Tina and drew a picture on the whiteboard of a mountain and a trail winding back and forth to reach the top.

"Have you ever been on a hike up a mountain?" I asked her.

"No," she said, "but I have been on some hikes that were really long."

"Good," I said, "so you get the idea. The path that we are setting out on is a long one. It will involve two separate procedures and two separate doses of anesthesia. It will require you to recover from one procedure and then have another one in a week or so. There are risks involved in both procedures. I am confident that we can get you to the top of this mountain, but it may seem like a long journey for someone your age. Do you understand?"

"Yes," she said.

At the initial consultation, I had asked Tammy if she and

her husband were raising Tina with a faith or religion. "No," she had replied, and Tina quickly added, "But we have a Christmas tree." I never want to make people feel awkward, but you have to do the best for the patient. I knew I had the training and skills to do the procedure successfully; I had previously treated tumors like the one behind her face. However, I wanted to offer Tina more; I wanted to offer her prayer. This time, my heart was pounding. It would have been easier to proceed had there not been a Harvard doctor in the room who already probably thought my colleagues and I were inferior to the surgeons he knew in the Northeast.

"It is my habit to pray with patients," I said boldly. "Would it be okay if I prayed for Tina?"

Richard looked at Tammy. Both looked surprised. She nodded yes and looked down at the floor. Dr. Willard stood up.

"I will wait in the waiting room," he said as he grasped the door handle and walked out. Clearly, he wanted no part in the prayer. I swallowed hard but moved ahead with what I felt was the best for the girl. It took some courage, given Dr. Willard's response. I moved over to Tina and put my hand on her shoulder.

"God, thank you for Tina," I prayed. "You invite us to ask you for what we want, and I am asking for your help and for success for both of the surgeries without any damage to Tina. Please give peace to her and her parents. In Jesus' name, Amen."

Tina seemed intrigued by the new experience and not apprehensive in the least. Tammy wiped tears from her eyes.

With a feeling of sobriety and expectation I stood and walked them to the waiting room where Dr. Willard was. I would see them the following day.

Early the next morning I went into the pre-op area to see Tina and her mother. Tammy exclaimed, "I had a dream last night that the tumor was gone." I smiled at the hope in her voice. When I examined Tina's face, I shook my head. It was still swollen where the tumor was: she would need the two long surgeries. I held her hand and Tammy's, said a quick prayer, and the transportation team wheeled Tina into surgery.

I put on my blue two-piece lead suit and a neck collar to protect me from radiation "scatter" while working with the X-rays. Donning a surgical hat and mask, I entered the procedure room where Tina lay unconscious, draped in a blue cloth with only a small patch of skin exposed over the femoral artery. She was lying on a table attached to a multimillion dollar, computerized machine that was necessary to see with detail through the skull and into the brain vessels. Two technologists were there, one dressed in a sterile gown and gloves to assist me, and one running the machine and opening supplies for us from the back table as needed. The anesthesiologist sat on the other side of the table behind leaded glass.

I felt for a pulse in Tina's femoral artery as it crossed her hip. As usual, I paused for a moment to remind myself that this was a person and not a project, which is easy to forget in a sterile environment. "God, keep her safe," I said before placing a long, hollow needle in her leg. We enter this artery because it travels over the femoral head, a large bone that allows compression of the puncture site after the procedure. The carotid artery in the neck is closer to the brain, but compression of the neck to seal the entry site after the procedure is more difficult and dangerous.

The red blood dripped rapidly back from the needle, indicating that I was in the artery. I inserted a wire through the hollow needle, then pulled out the needle and slid over the wire a tapered plastic tube or sheath, like a drinking straw with a narrow pointed tip and a one-way valve on the end. One of the techs handed me the sterile catheter and guidewire. I slid it through the one-way valve in Tina's leg and began the journey through the vessels to the tumor in her head.

Endovascular neurosurgery is surprisingly tactile. With your fingers you insert a guidewire, less than one millimeter in diameter, and a two-millimeter guide catheter into the femoral artery. By hand, you gently push these up toward the heart, with the guide catheter sliding up over the wire in coaxial fashion. Feeding the wire involves fine finger movements, not unlike those used in sewing or spindle work. None of it is done by machine. The guidewire has a curve on the tip and can be directed into different vessels by rotating it. If you feel resistance, you have to stop and figure out why. All movement must be calculated; extra or exaggerated movement is dangerous. Experience tells you what kind of resistance you are meeting as you watch the wire move through the body.

I gently pushed the guidewire and the guide catheter against the flow of blood coming down from Tina's heart. Within moments I reached the top of her aortic arch, where three main vessels branch off to the neck, face, and head. I had gone against the flow of blood coming up from the leg, and now I would go with the flow to the head.

Across Tina's body from me during the procedure were several large screens. When I stepped on the floor pedal, the machine would come to life and show a live image of the field of interest. I watched on the screen as X-rays flowed where I directed them and Tina's gray, beating heart became visible between her white, air-filled lungs. The metal wire was black against the gray background. We always check carefully for air bubbles in the lines and in the contrast dye we inject. Anything injected from this point will flow into the brain, which pulls in blood like a vacuum. I knew in advance which of the three branches led to the tumor. From three feet away, I rotated the guidewire and watched on the screen as it flipped up and into the carotid artery. There was a sense of accomplishment at every step. All this was done by feel and by knowing where the different arteries branched off the aortic arch.

The procedure was going well, and I was thankful that Tina was young. The older that people are, the more tortuous their vessels can be and the more difficult it is to get to where you want to go. You can struggle for more than an hour just getting the guide catheter in place, as I had done with Daniel. Arteriosclerosis, calcification, and a general slanting of the vessels with age make them curvy and difficult to navigate. These factors also make it dangerous to straighten out the vessels with your instruments because this can break plaque off the sides, which can travel to the brain and cause a stroke. Young, malleable vessels are much easier to work in, and Tina's vessels remained beautifully flexible.

The first goal with any endovascular neurosurgery is to get the guide catheter situated properly in the carotid artery in the neck. This becomes the "base camp" from which I enter the brain, or in this case, the face, with an even smaller tube called a micro-catheter. Endovascular surgery is like virtual reality surgery. It is performed with the aid of continual X-rays that show the field of operation. Wires, balloons, and stents all have metal markers so that they show up under X-ray.

The X-ray machine and contrast dye that are needed to see into the vessels are costly, not just financially but physically. Contrast dye is harmful to the kidneys and must be used sparingly, especially in a child. Every time I step on the machine's pedal to see inside the body, the patient and parts of the doctor are radiated. Radiation is harmful, and I've heard estimates that 2 percent of all cancer cases will soon be caused by radiation given in hospitals for tests and procedures. Therefore, you must balance your need for updated information (gained with contrast and radiation) against doing the best you can with the information you have. In a long case with a high radiation dose, the patient can actually experience hair loss and skin irritation in the area where the X-ray beam passes through the head. Though the hair grows back within six months, radiation has a powerful, damaging effect, and it is not to be unleashed lightly.

As well as Tina's surgery had been going, there was still

no guarantee of the desired outcome. From the moment you enter the artery in the leg, things can go wrong. The artery is made up of three layers, and it is possible to cause dissections through the vessel layers—tears in the soft, slippery inner lining, laying open the muscular layer underneath. A vessel dissection can allow blood clots to form on the rough muscular layer, which can then break off and cause a stroke. You are always navigating between the dangers of causing bleeding or causing clotting. Both lead to stroke. In addition, you are never sure how the body will respond to the invasiveness of a catheter running half the length of the body through a major artery. The artery can spasm around the catheter, cutting off blood flow to the brain on that side. It is possible for a catheter navigated far out in the circulation to be stuck and unable to be removed after glue injections. The longer you are inside the vessels with your instruments, the higher the chances of something going wrong.

I guided the micro-catheter using a micro-guidewire, positioning them in a feeding vessel to the tumor in Tina's face. Once I was certain that I was in the optimal position, I pushed a liquid embolizing agent into the tumor's blood supply to close it. This took more than six hours of concentration because of the size of the tumor and the generous blood supply it was receiving from the internal carotid artery and the ophthalmic artery. It was slow and tedious work, with many stressful moments when I had to make snap decisions about how aggressively to fill the critical areas with blocking agent—arteries that went directly to Tina's eye and brain. Finally, I believed that I had accomplished what I had set out to do.

After the procedure, I waited for Tina to wake up. I was exhausted from the procedure and had just one desire: to know Tina was okay. After thirty minutes or so that felt like hours, Tina awoke. I held up fingers in front of her face, and she counted them perfectly. She had sight in both eyes and was able to move both arms and legs. It appeared that after many hours of painstaking work, she had suffered no neurological deficits.

Dr. Willard, Tammy, and Richard were in the waiting room, anxious after the seven-hour wait. I told them things had gone well and showed them a picture of the tumor, which was now obviously filled with the agent and cut off from its blood supply. Dr. Willard looked at the scans and seemed pleased. Several days later, Tina had open surgery, which was done by our outstanding skull base team, consisting of another neurosurgeon and a head and neck surgeon. The entire tumor was removed with very little blood loss. The liquid embolizing agent had cut off the blood supply, the open surgery was a success, and Tina went home a few days later. After six weeks her facial incisions were barely visible.

I received a card from Tammy a month after the surgery. She thanked me again for the special care that Tina had received. Six months later, I was surprised to receive a letter from Dr. Willard:

Dear Dr. Levy,

It is hard to find words to express my heartfelt gratitude for you and the team for the exceptionally competent care that you provided my granddaughter, Tina, during her recent bout with a stage 4 tumor. From my first meeting with you in preparation for Tina's embolization, I was especially impressed with your caring manner and that rare ability to relate to this young child who was about to endure such a horrific and complex set of medical and surgical procedures. You were able to help Tina and her parents clearly understand what treatment was necessary and openly face the serious risks that were involved.

After forty years in the medical profession I have rarely experienced such a profound combination of clinical, personable, and spiritual competence in one physician.

As a result, your words, manner, and spiritual input put Tina's frightened parents at ease and left them with a sense of hope. For this our family will ever be grateful.[1]

When I read that letter, I remembered the courage it had required for me to pray in front of a physician who had spent his career at some of the best hospitals in the world. I was glad I hadn't shied away from caring for Tina in the best way I knew how, which was by addressing the whole person.

As happy as I was with the results of praying with patients, I had still feared praying in front of other medical professionals. It was a fear that took a great deal of courage to overcome—and that finally reached a breaking point.

CHAPTER 5

FACING MY COLLEAGUES

PRAYER HAD BECOME A COMFORTABLE PART of my routine. Patient reactions were overwhelmingly positive, and I even felt prayer was improving the outcomes of the procedures. Still, though, I was confining my prayers to those brief times when I was alone with the patient before and after surgery. I was afraid to pray in the presence of anyone who was not the patient or family. Mostly, this meant the nurses.

Nurses are powerful and extremely valuable members of the hospital staff; no hospital can be first-rate without good ones. Nurses can make a huge difference in a patient's stay and in a doctor's day. Good nurses know their patients well and can often point out things a doctor may miss. They notice what goes on in the operating room and even whose patients have the most complications after surgery. I value and need their opinions, assessments, and care in a hectic environment, so I wondered what they would think of me for potentially violating their sense of decorum in the medical setting.

If a nurse makes one subtle, negative comment regarding a doctor, within seconds that doctor's standing, at least among the nurses, can be devastated, rightly or wrongly. Of course they still have to follow his orders; they just don't respect him. It probably shouldn't matter to us, but deep inside, every doctor is keenly aware of his reputation and afraid of losing the respect of those around him. The idea that nurses might pass judgment on you and that this opinion might somehow percolate up to your own colleagues is threatening, no matter how you try to ignore or minimize it.

I was living with fear and double-mindedness. Even though I was praying with patients, I did not want to be known as someone who prayed with patients. I was certain the nurses and other doctors would misunderstand my motivation and would even question my integrity as a surgeon. To make it more challenging, I had been working at the hospital for seven years and had formed long-term relationships there. People had a pretty good sense of who I was. To introduce this radical change in behavior could destabilize these relationships and attract attention and questions I just didn't want to deal with.

But praying in secret was proving unbearably frustrating. Waiting for the nurses and the anesthesia personnel to leave the room so I could pray was easily the most miserable part of my day. I was bound up in anxiety each time I was forced to wait. I couldn't count the number of times I lurked around pre-op, killing time or pretending to read a chart in a patient's bay while waiting for nurses to finish their work and head off to other tasks.

Then I was brought to a point of decision.

I walked into the busy pre-operative area one day feeling that mixture of hopeful anticipation and frustration. I was looking forward to praying, as usual, but not to waiting for all the nurses and anesthesiologists to clear out. In spite of my best efforts I had found no reliable way to time my entrance to see the patient alone. I had tried arriving early, but the administrative personnel were often there placing the hospital wristband. I had tried arriving late, but the anesthesiologist was often there. During the rest of the time, the nurses were ever present. If I came too late, I would miss my chance because the transportation team would be carting the patient off to the procedure room.

On this day I stood there, trying to look busy while waiting for the industrious nurse to leave. My level of irritation kept rising. I felt impatient, anxious, out of control. Suddenly, an inner voice—I knew it was God—posed an unexpected and simple question: "Do you believe that what you are doing, praying before surgery, is a good thing?"

I thought about it a moment, then answered silently, "Yes,

I know it is good. I have seen the effects of prayer in calmed nerves and tears of emotional release, and I have heard the patients' reports."

"Then why are you afraid? If you don't believe in what you are doing, why don't you stop doing it?"

That got my attention. Stop praying? I couldn't do that. I had opened up a whole other avenue of care that was blessing people and blessing me. Praying was now something I enjoyed. I didn't want to stop; I just wanted to continue in secret.

"I can't stop praying," I answered. "It wouldn't be right for me or for them."

"Then why are you afraid?" the voice persisted.

I had to answer truthfully: I was afraid because I still valued what people would think or say about me and my reputation.

Stung, I argued back, "But I don't want people to think that I'm one of those weirdos who go around praying for people. Good grief, I've worked for years to build a reputation in my field and in this hospital."

"You don't want to be known as someone who goes around praying for people?" the voice asked.

"That's right," I answered silently.

"But you do go around praying for people, don't you?" the voice asked, and even though no one else could have heard our conversation, I actually turned red with shame.

"Yes, but I don't want people thinking that I do!" was all I could respond.

It was clear to me that God was calling me out for my lack of authenticity.

I wanted to have it both ways—to pray for people and see the power and comfort that it brought them but not to be thought of as someone who prayed for people or believed that God is relevant to medical care. To stop living that lie would take courage, but it would also provide relief if I could do it—no more waiting around for nurses to leave, no more agonizing or hiding my actions. I saw before me the tantalizing freedom that would come from being bold and single minded. I also saw the risks to my reputation and to my pride.

I had a choice to make.

In that moment, with the pre-op activities buzzing around me, I decided to step into authenticity no matter what it cost me—my reputation, my job, or the respect of my coworkers. Swallowing whatever resistance my heart still offered, I walked up to the foot of my patient's bed.

"Good morning, Mrs. Greene," I said.

"Good morning, Doctor," she replied. She looked weary and resigned, as if a long journey had brought her to this moment. The nurse patiently swabbed her arm, acknowledging neither of us.

"You and I have talked about the surgery you're about to undergo. You understand the risks involved," I said.

"Yes, I do," Mrs. Greene said.

"This morning I will be going in to fix the aneurysm in the back of your brain. If it goes well, you'll be out and recovering in a couple of hours. Are there any other questions you have for me at this time?"

"No, I don't think so," she said.

Without allowing myself to pause, for fear that I might stop altogether, I continued, "Then is it okay if I say a prayer for you?"

I knew the reaction was coming.

I saw the nurse sitting with her back to me, bent over Mrs. Greene's left arm so that I couldn't see it, preparing her for an IV. The nurse stopped what she was doing, glanced at me quickly, and sat up straight. She said nothing. Mrs. Greene looked at me askance, too, then nodded.

"Okay," she said, seeming a bit distracted.

Without hesitation, I grabbed her toes through the blanket and began to pray.

"God, I thank you for Mrs. Greene. She is precious to you, and I ask for wisdom and skill to fix her vessels. We ask you for success. Give her peace now. Amen."

When I opened my eyes, I expected to see a peaceful expression gracing Mrs. Greene's face, as I had seen on dozens of other faces. Instead she looked uncomfortable and was trying to smile through obvious pain. Looking in the direction of the nurse and Mrs. Greene's arm, I realized that in my determination to pray I had not paid attention to what was happening procedurally. The nurse had put the IV needle into Mrs. Greene's arm and was searching for a vein as I had made my offer to pray. She had stopped her work out of reverence and automatically bowed her head when I began praying, leaving the needle hanging out of the patient's arm the whole time. No wonder Mrs. Greene was having trouble concentrating.

Fumbling with my words, I apologized that I had interrupted this delicate routine. The nurse resumed her hunt for the vein, found it, and taped the needle to Mrs. Greene's arm.

"Thank you," Mrs. Greene said to both of us with evident relief.

Though I had bungled the timing, I had also crossed a threshold of courage and was determined not to turn back. I still preferred to pray with the patient and family alone, because it was simpler. I considered it a sacred and beautiful moment, and I did not want to have it lessened for my patients by having others present who might not value the moment the same way. Neither did I want to worry about offending or inconveniencing the nurses or other health care professionals, but from that point on I was able to pray in front of nurses if necessary. Over the next few months I steeled myself many times and prayed in their presence. I earned a number of shocked looks. *What is this doctor doing?* they seemed to be thinking. *This is something new. Wait till the others hear about this.* Many of them would stop working long enough to let the prayer pass, like a gust of wind. Some bowed their heads and seemed to participate silently. Others kept working as if nothing were happening.

Their reactions still mattered to me, but it mattered more that I was being authentic and doing what I thought was best for my patients, even if others thought it foolish. Courage had taken me further down the path of authenticity.

• • •

A few months later I was in the room of a particular patient who was about to undergo surgery to repair a massive tangle of vessels that had improperly formed in his brain. I did my normal pre-op talk. The nurse was heading out to get something, but when I asked the patient if I could pray, the nurse made a U-turn and came back quietly. Her shoulder-length black hair hung partially over her face as she bowed her head. The two family members and I held hands with the patient. The nurse stood behind us and listened during the short prayer.

When we had finished and I turned to leave the pre-op area, the nurse stepped into my path and pulled me aside.

"Dr. Levy?"

"Yes?" I responded, thinking, *Probably a curbside consult*— a doctors' term for when a nurse or anyone else approaches you in the hallway or elevator to ask advice about a loved one with a medical issue. This is almost the only time nurses approach doctors outside a professional context. I did not know this nurse by name, and she was clearly nervous. She avoided my eyes and wrung her hands. It gave me a chance to see "Cheryl" on her name badge.

"The other nurses and I have noticed that you pray for people," Cheryl said. This wasn't what I was expecting, and I felt my stomach do a quick flip.

"Yes," I said, bracing myself for whatever was next. Cheryl shifted from one foot to another, hesitant to come to her purpose.

"I want to join you next time. Would you call me when you are about to pray?" she said, then continued in a hushed voice. "There are other nurses who want to be in on that too. Would you include us?"

I was amazed. Yet again, the thing that I feared would bring division and mockery had instead drawn people in. The nurses had indeed talked about what I was doing—but not in the way I had expected. Perhaps my actions had offered another care option to some who had not considered it before. Clearly, some of them wanted to be part of something more than just fixing people's bodies—like me, they wanted to bless patients, body and soul.

"Sure," I said. "I'll look for you."

"Thank you," Cheryl said and had the courage to look me in the eye briefly before walking back to the desk.

After that, I began to invite some of the nurses who expressed interest to join the prayers. Often they had to take off their latex gloves or stop what they were doing (especially if they had been about to place an IV), but many seemed eager to join in.

This is another area in which to proceed very delicately, and I am sensitive to allow nurses to say no if they wish. I have to be careful not to misuse the authority and responsibility I have as the lead physician. It would be wrong to compel a nurse to pray, just as it would be wrong to compel a patient to pray. I choose my phrasing carefully and make sure my tone is welcoming but not commanding. I have never heard a complaint from a nurse. Some continue working as if uninterested, but some are actually quite animated and will even add an "Amen" of their own.

Once I became open to including nurses if they desired, the unity of the pre-op prayer experience suddenly seemed complete. I had learned early on that when some people pray, they like to hold hands and "circle up." Some families did this automatically when I prayed for the patient, and soon I began to encourage family members to hold the patient's hand and one another's. The act of forming a circle gave us a strong sense of unity unlike anything I had experienced in a medical setting. Brothers and sisters who hadn't gotten along would come together and unite around someone they loved, reminding them of what was truly important. Family from far away would draw in close. Prayer united us all in our desire to see a successful surgery for the person we cared about.

Now the nurses are sometimes part of those prayer circles. Certainly I always knew that most nurses truly care about their patients, but their occasional willingness to join those pre-operative prayers adds a warmth and collegial spirit that is unique in my experience.

The nurses' response was more than I could have wished for. But that wasn't the end of my road to authenticity—there was more to come.

• • •

I was offering to pray with patients before and after each surgery. The habit had breathed life into my practice and into the lives of those around me. Wherever prayer happened, the atmosphere often changed for the better, and I became convinced that I should be praying at every juncture of every procedure. That necessarily brought me to the next threshold of bravery: praying in front of those who help me in surgery.

It was one thing to pray in front of nurses; we see each other for only a few minutes each week. There is another group of people, however, with whom I work daily, who know me much better and whose opinions matter more to me—the technologists, the people who spend hours helping me during the actual surgeries.

Technologists work with X-rays. They are not doctors, but they are highly trained specialists. Their career paths usually start with taking basic X-rays of the hand or foot; if they choose, they can train to assist in interventional procedures in the body or brain. The team of seven techs with whom I had worked for seven years by this time are my extra sets of hands during surgery. They prepare and hand me the delicate instruments and run the multimillion dollar, computerized imaging system that allows me to do the work in the brain. They have come to know how I operate, the types of devices and mixtures I prefer, and when I usually take pictures during a procedure—not to mention the tone of my voice, how quickly I work, how I react to stress, and what I am likely to do when we reach an impasse. We are a tight, battle-tested team. I not only know them by name, I know their histories and their families. Our intimacy befits the seriousness of the procedures we tackle together.

To introduce prayer into our shared routine would be my biggest step yet because it would change a long-standing relationship into which we all had invested a good deal of trust. However, by this time I was more confident than I had been in the past, and more resolved. I knew there was still the possibility that my team members would react poorly to prayer and might even reject me personally, but that wasn't going to stop me from at least asking. I could no longer deny that there was more than technology and chance at play in our procedures. For years we had never acknowledged that our work had a spiritual component, even when aneurysms ruptured and people died on the table before our eyes. Now I had seen the effects of prayer and believed that God helps those who ask—how could I keep pretending that all success was due to my skills or to blind luck? Ultimately, I believed prayer was the best thing for my patients, but did I have the boldness to ask God to affect outcomes in front of others?

Before every procedure, the techs and I gather in the reading room, a small five-by-ten space with backlit panels on one wall to hang the X-rays and a tall computer screen that depicts the brain in 3-D rendering. You can rotate the image of the brain in any direction using a trackball. There we discuss the day's procedures in detail before heading in to perform the surgery.

On the day I decided to pray, techs Jeff and Heather were there along with a sales rep from a medical device company. We discussed the aneurysm shape and the vessels leading to it. I had my own ideas, but that day I asked for everyone's opinion on which devices to use for the repair. Of course we expected the medical device representative to recommend his devices, and he did. When I couldn't think of another angle to bring up about the case, and I could feel my heart pounding with anxiety, I simply said, "I would like to say a prayer for this patient before we begin. I need to ask you all if you are comfortable with that. I respect the relationship that I have with each of you, and it is very important that I not coerce or force you. You don't need to stay for this."

All three of them stood there not saying a word, absorbing the new wrinkle in their routine and perhaps wondering if I had lost my mind. Then they seemed to give a collective shrug, as if to say, "Whatever." They didn't know what to do while I prayed; they just stared at the floor. It was awkward for all of us, but nobody left.

"Heavenly Father," I said, "we thank you for our jobs and that we have the opportunity to fix this aneurysm on Mr. Simmons. We ask for your wisdom on what to do and when to stop. Thank you for Jeff and Heather, and bless them with keen eyes and ears as they help in this case. Please bless their families this week. Give us joy as we do the surgery today. In Jesus' name, Amen."

With that, we entered the procedure room and did our jobs, while acting as though nothing unusual had occurred. The next week I did the same thing, and nearly every case thereafter. Nothing immediately changed in our relationships. Nobody protested, even though some were members of other religions or of no religion at all. Over the ensuing weeks I noticed that I had more joy during the procedures, and it seemed that we were having fewer complications. I saw the staff exhibit greater care and humanity toward the patients and toward one another. They saw that I took faith seriously but that I did not judge them. Talking to God was not some empty ritual but something active and alive.

Still, I wondered what they really thought about this new habit. Maybe they were resigned to working with an eccentric surgeon, or maybe they didn't want to lose favor with me. I soon saw it was more than that. One day I went in to an emergency procedure and was so rushed that I forgot to pray. I had put on my gown and gloves and was approaching the table where a teenage boy was lying. Lydia, whose long hair was tucked under a blue surgical cap, came between me and the table.

"We need to pray," she reminded me.

Of all the techs to say this, she might be the one some would least expect. Lydia was an attractive woman with a big heart toward vulnerable patients. She was also living a lifestyle many religious people would find offensive. And she loved praying before procedures. Behind her safety glasses, there was a serious look in her eyes that let me know she was not pretending. She had a genuine concern for the patient. She really wanted me to pray.

"You're right," I said beneath my mask. I grabbed her sterile-gloved hand in mine and touched the patient through sterile draping with my other hand.

"God, be with this boy," I prayed, as Lydia closed her eyes and touched his blue-draped leg with her other hand. "Give us wisdom and skill. Keep us alert and aware of things we need to know to do this well. In Jesus' name, Amen."

We opened our eyes and looked up at each other. There was a certain sparkle and assurance in her gaze. I felt better. God was strengthening us as individuals and as a team through this simple act of prayer.

Some weeks later one of the other techs, Heather, cornered me while I was in the reading room dictating a case. She sat down, looking at me strangely.

"Something has happened to you over the years," she said. "I can see it. You're different than you were."

"Am I?" I answered noncommittally.

"Tell me about your faith," she said. "How did it happen? Did you come to it suddenly?"

I stopped what I was doing.

"It was gradual," I said, and I explained a little about how I had discovered that there was much more to life than using my gifts for my own glory and financial gain—that life could have a greater purpose, but you had to make the effort to pursue it.

Heather was quiet for a while.

"My husband lost his job," she said finally, tearing up.

"I'm sorry to hear that," I said. She waved it off professionally, but with evident emotion.

"For the first time in our marriage we prayed together last night," Heather said. "I thought you would want to know."

"I'm glad to hear that," I said, feeling a swell of joy. "How did it feel?"

"It felt great. We needed it," Heather sighed.

"I am really proud of you—I hope you will continue," I encouraged.

She nodded in agreement.

"We all really appreciate it when you pray before procedures," she told me, and in the pause that ensued, I could sense that she wanted more than just conversation; she wanted some sort of help.

"Do you mind if I pray for your situation right now?" I offered.

"Sure. Go ahead," she said, exhaling.

"Heavenly Father, you know Heather and you know Bruce," I said. "You know the financial struggles that they're going through at this time. I know that you have good things planned for them in the future, because you are good. Bruce needs wisdom right now to make the best decisions for his career and family. I ask for a blessing on them even this week, something special so that they would know it is from you. In Jesus' name, Amen."

I looked up. She was wiping away tears. The same peace that pervaded the reading room in the mornings when we prayed was here this afternoon, flooding her heart. She had moved toward God, the source of that peace.

A short time later Bruce decided to make a career change, returning to school to become a medical technologist. This proved to be a positive breakthrough for them. After that,

Heather and Bruce found a church they enjoyed and began taking more steps to know God.

• • •

The next hurdle for me was praying with my fellow M.D.s. I had few opportunities to pray with other physicians, and I was not looking for them. Of all the groups in the hospital setting, I most feared judgment from other doctors.

Occasionally I am called on by device manufacturers to train others in the use of new medical devices. One week I traveled to a hospital in another city to teach two physicians, one of whom I knew to be a Muslim and the other a Hindu, to use a new intracranial stent for complex aneurysms. I was a proctor, essentially a consultant, observing and adding the extra information and experience they would need to use the device correctly on a human being.

I was not even sure that the patient in this case knew I was involved. I didn't intend to interact with her or address her. I would merely be present in the procedure room while she was undergoing the operation and give suggestions from the back of the room. However, when the other physicians and I huddled on the morning of the procedure, they unexpectedly asked me to accompany them to see her in pre-op. Somewhat reluctantly, I walked with them to her bedside.

"This is the doctor we've told you about," they said proudly.

"Oh, from San Diego. I've heard all about you," she said.

Dottie, an Australian, was fifty but looked sixty-five because of her two-pack-a-day smoking habit. She had a complex aneurysm that required a stent, the device I would be teaching them to use. We smiled and shook hands, but I felt a tightening on the inside. Now that Dottie knew I was involved as the expert, I felt I had a greater responsibility to her. I needed to offer to pray for her because that's what I did for all my patients.

The problem was these two other doctors. How would I introduce prayer when it wasn't my patient and wasn't even my hospital? How would they react, being from different religions? Was prayer appropriate in this context where I was simply teaching others to use a medical device? I had so many unanswered questions; surely I could make an exception in this case and not pray. It was too uncomfortable. Surely God would understand and let me off on a technicality.

As we made small talk with Dottie for a minute, I wondered what to do. I felt vulnerable. For me to assert something like this in someone else's hospital would take another level of courage.

So I stalled, hoping that the other doctors would find some reason to leave me alone with her—not likely. Then, as I extended the small talk past its normal duration, the words *head and shoulders* flashed into my mind. *Head & Shoulders?* I asked myself. *What does dandruff shampoo have to do with this situation?* Then I thought of that part of the Bible where Saul was anointed king of Israel. It says that he stood head and shoulders taller than his fellow countrymen in terms of height, but when it was his time to shine at his coronation party, they found him hiding among the baggage.[1] That was me, hiding among the baggage. I felt that God was telling me that as their teacher, I was in a position of honor. Professionally speaking, my experience was much greater, and I did not need to hide myself or my special treatment of patients from them.

That was enough for me. I knew that I at least needed to offer to pray for her. I looked at Dottie, smiled, and forced the words out.

"It is my custom to pray with patients before surgery," I said to her. "Do you mind if I pray with you?"

Dottie looked at me curiously. "All right," she said.

I grabbed her hand. The other doctors had fallen silent. My words seemed to have frozen them in place—they stood fixed and staring at the floor. When I bowed my head, they quickly bowed theirs.

"Gracious God," I began, and I prayed for the success of her surgery. When the prayer was over, the other doctors came back to life but didn't know what to say. Dottie smiled quizzically, as though she'd just been given a gift she didn't know what to do with. After a moment she said, with that wonderful Aussie accent, "Thank you. I've never heard of a doctor praying before."

I bet these other two docs have never heard of it either, I thought.

My colleagues were much less conversational as we walked out and prepared for the surgery. To break the silence, I brought up a technical aspect of the case, which put them very much at ease as we walked down the stairs. Prayer was simply part of my approach. Indeed, I was teaching something that I hadn't intended.

We performed two surgeries that day, and both went well. The Muslim doctor had to be elsewhere for the second one, leaving me with Rajiv, the Hindu doctor. Again, we visited a patient in pre-op in need of a brain stent. This time I did not hesitate to ask to pray. The patient agreed, and I grabbed his hand. Before I knew what was happening, Rajiv walked to the other side of the gurney and grabbed the patient's other hand. He then reached for my hand, which I gave him, and we formed a small prayer circle. My colleague clenched his eyes shut and waited for me to pray. What a joy it was to see that Rajiv, typically reserved, wanted to be on the inside this time, part of whatever was taking place in the spiritual realm. When we finished, he was smiling and much more at ease than before. He was even jovial as we walked out. We both acted as if nothing of consequence had occurred, but I noticed a certain levity as we discussed the technical aspects of the next case.

That experience liberated me further. There are always new challenges and obstacles. No matter how many times I have prayed, I remain conscious that my offer may be offensive to some. It still takes courage when any new person is added to the mix—a visiting doctor or medical student, for example. I simply announce that it is my habit to pray before surgery and ask if that is okay with everyone, and I look at each person for his or her response. Almost everyone says it is.

By degrees, my profession was becoming bigger than the technical aspect of my cases. Prayer in support of my neurosurgery practice was becoming my calling. This was a long way from where I had started.

CHAPTER 6

FROM MECHANIC
TO MEDICAL SCHOOL

IT'S NOT UNUSUAL for surgeons to talk about the "mechanics" of the work we do, but I am the only neurosurgeon I know who actually began his career working on cars.

The idea of being a doctor didn't enter my mind as a young man. In high school I had no goals or motivation and made little effort at my studies. I did only what came easily. My parents were pretty sure I would do poorly in college, so they suggested that I instead look into a school for auto mechanics. I shrugged off even that modest goal because I could already fix cars and was in fact working as a gas station attendant. Nothing in my life said "higher degree," much less "medical school" or "brain surgery."

Then one day my older brother, who had gone to work on an oil rig off the coast of Louisiana, mentioned that the "college boys" on the rig seemed to have easier jobs that didn't involve grease up to their elbows. They made more money and got to boss around those who hadn't gone to college. That caught my attention. Then my aunt sent enough money for me to take one class at the local college. About this time I had started dreaming of being an actor, so I decided to get a college degree as a fallback plan, then work on an oil rig until I made enough money to buy a motorcycle and ride to Hollywood, where I would begin my true career on the silver screen. Real practical.

In the meantime I was working at the gas station and tire shop with the station owner's son. One day there was a lull in the action, and we were leaning on the gas pumps talking. He told me he was taking the MCAT—Medical College Admission Test—and hoped to go to medical school. It was the first time I had heard of someone actually preparing to be a doctor—the first time I understood there was a pathway toward that kind of career. I didn't think much of it, but later that week I had something akin to an epiphany. My car was making a funny noise when I shifted gears, so I got underneath it and started taking apart the transmission. As I held one of the parts in my grease-covered hands, it occurred to me: if I could fix cars, I could fix people. The idea of repairing a "machine" as complex as the human body captivated me.

Two years later I was admitted to medical school.

At twenty years of age, I was the youngest person in my

class at medical school and desperate for a sense of identity and belonging. David Levy is a very Jewish name, and I rather looked forward to the distinction of being a "Jewish doctor."

My father, Isaac Levy, was a Sephardic Jew by birth and was raised in an Orthodox Jewish family. Previously, the family had lost their home and business under Nazi persecution. My well-to-do grandparents left everything on the island of Rhodes to escape Hitler's stranglehold on Europe and eventually made it to the United States. The more than 1,600 Jews who didn't leave the island were taken to concentration camps. Many of them died.

As a young adult my father accepted Jesus as the Jewish Messiah and was promptly ostracized by his family and community. The experience was painful for him, but he found meaning and purpose in both the Hebrew Scriptures and the New Testament, which came alive to him. My dad had experienced two kinds of persecution. He had been persecuted for being a Jew; then persecuted by Jews for believing in Jesus. I think for that reason he almost never talked about his past. I knew very little about my Jewish heritage except for the yearly Passover our family celebrated. Perhaps wanting to protect us from the rejection he faced, he settled in a small town so we grew up with no Jewish friends and little exposure to our heritage. I had no idea what Jewish culture was.

From the time I was young, I regarded Jesus as special. Knowing that my father endured persecution because of his decision to follow Jesus, I respected his beliefs. I dutifully learned the stories from the Old and New Testaments. I wanted to believe the stories of Jesus walking on water, healing people, forgiving sins, and rising from the dead. With a heroic Savior like Jesus, who had sacrificed himself to pay for my sins so that I could have a relationship with a holy and benevolent God, the world seemed to make more sense. Then I went to medical school.

Suddenly I found that Jews made up a third of my classmates, which was something of a culture shock to me. Having had little exposure to Jewish people before, I was pleasantly surprised to find them truly engaging. They were wealthy and witty, they loved to laugh and seemed to really enjoy life, they drove nice cars—and the Jewish women were beautiful. What more could a twenty-year-old guy want? It felt wonderful to belong. Besides, I dreamed of discovering a cure for cancer or stroke—some significant accomplishment that would change the world and inspire love and admiration on top of it. It seemed that Jewish doctors had accomplished much in medicine, and I wanted to belong to this group.

I also appreciated the contrast with the Christian culture I had known in small-town America. The Christians there were often poor and struggling, and had irritating and legalistic personalities. They were always bringing long lists of problems to God, with mixed results. They seemed impoverished and powerless to help themselves. How refreshing it was to finally be with people who had the money, the power, and the energy to make life work.

I fully embraced a heritage I had never known. I went

with friends to synagogue. I felt self-righteous when I would fast on Yom Kippur (the Day of Atonement) and eat matzo (unleavened bread) during the seven days of Passover. I sat through services in Hebrew, a language most of us didn't understand. Only once, out of curiosity, did I attend a Christian function near campus, and then a Jewish class-mate heard about it and questioned me. After that, I never went again for fear of what people in my new community would say.

The Jewish culture is something for which I gained the tremendous respect that I hold to this day. I liked this feeling of community as I sat in the synagogue on the Jewish High Holy Days, but by my fourth year in medical school, I began to feel conflicted. Deep within I couldn't deny that Jesus was special, but I didn't want him to be God or Messiah to me. I didn't want to worship Jesus. In my view, he was too humble, too nice, and too easily walked on. That wasn't who I wanted to be. Besides, in the halls of higher education, there didn't seem to be much need for God or Jesus. I was learning that medicine and surgery had the power to save lives—and that power would soon be mine. Following Jesus seemed so dull and boring compared to the public acclaim, fun, and excitement available to me as a Jew—and as a doctor.

While I lacked social confidence among my classmates, who were two years older, I had virtually unlimited technical confidence. It was in the third year of medical school that I began to come into my element. Having focused mostly on book learning until that point, now our studies afforded us direct contact with patients in order to learn how to treat their ailments. I discovered how much I enjoyed the procedural side of medicine—and that I was good at it. Now I was determined to excel at it.

One of my first goals was to learn how to put in a central line, something typically learned during the first year of medical/surgical residency, two years in the future for me. Placing a central line, the first seriously risky procedure that a resident learns, is a big step up from starting a standard IV. It involves placing a three-inch-long needle under the clavicle into the large vein that resides there. Puncturing the top of the lung is the most feared risk, and it can be fatal if not recognized. Because human anatomy varies, finding this vein is a little like drilling for oil. As a third-year medical student, I had watched demonstrations, but it was unlikely that anyone would allow me to place a central line. Unless, of course, there was an emergency.

If someone in a hospital stops breathing or has some other life-threatening condition, a Code Blue is called, and doctors and residents appear from all corners of the hospital to resuscitate the patient, which involves placing a central line. Medical students are supposed to watch. On my second Code Blue, I arrived quickly and there was nobody present to place the central line. I asked the nurse to hand me the central line kit. Taking in my short white coat, the distinguishing mark of a med student, she shook her head with contempt. A minute later a medical resident appeared, and she gave the kit to him. I tried asking for the kit on several other Code Blue episodes, with similar results.

This was standard hospital protocol, of course. Impatient at the thought of waiting another two years, however, I had my mother sew an extra pocket inside my lab coat, allowing me to carry a central line kit with me. Now when I heard a Code Blue being called over the hospital intercom, I would run up seven flights of stairs, pull out my own kit, and begin the procedure. After a quick swipe with an antiseptic prep, I would insert the three-inch needle under the patient's clavicle. I was a natural at procedures and relished the challenge. Confidence I had by the boatload. If a technique could be done, I knew I could master it. When I saw that dark blood flash into the syringe signaling that the needle was in the vein, I was elated—much to the consternation of the residents who arrived after I did. I would thread the line and flash an arrogant "Glad I was able to help" smile. I look back on this zeal for experience with some regret. By the grace of God, I was as able as I had thought—almost every attempt was successful, and no harm was done, except the alienation of my peers.

If there were other ways to get ahead, I seized them. I learned that writing scientific papers allowed me to go to meetings to present the papers, and that meant time off. It also meant the residency program would pay my way. Although writing papers during neurosurgical residency would be expected, doing so during my first-year, general-surgery internship was unusual—yet to the chagrin of my peers, I wrote several. The chief resident figured out that

I had more time away at meetings than he had, which did not sit well. In my naiveté, I actually thought that everyone else would be happy for me, like prisoners cheering one who breaks out. But nobody likes a guy who doesn't play by the unspoken rules. During the early years of the seven-year residency training, I used every opportunity to get ahead. If others didn't want to do that, could they blame me? That was my attitude. They could, and they did.

The later years of residency taught me to be a neurosurgeon. I grew in my appreciation for the teaching staff, which included some of the most highly respected neurosurgeons in the world. I developed bonds of collegiality and friendship with my coresidents as we strove together to perform at a level worthy of the profession we had chosen. Ambition to succeed and ambition to serve began to come into balance.

I became a neurosurgeon and went to Pennsylvania to accept a job that would allow me to practice open neurosurgery (opening the skull) as well as endovascular neurosurgery (accessing the brain through the vessels only). Because it was a busy practice, I had plenty of opportunities to operate and hone my skills. I also became much more concerned about the welfare of the patient than I had been during my training. Due to the large number of complex vascular diseases I encountered, my career was moving fast. I continued writing papers and technical notes, began taking speaking engagements, and traveling widely. I increased ever more in confidence and skill, and I planned to spend my life as one of the leaders in the field of academic neurosurgery.

I should have been the happiest guy in the world. My life was fast and entertaining, heroic and challenging. I had accomplished my dream. Yet something was not right. Though I had no lack of interest from beautiful women, including a fashion model I dated around that time, I couldn't keep a relationship alive. Everything seemed hollow. I noticed that I hated to be home and that I was traveling to avoid "normal" life. As time went on, I needed greater and more-complex cases to feel satisfied. At that time, I was at the forefront of the emerging, high-risk specialty that is endovascular neurosurgery. "Normal," day-to-day, standard neurosurgery left me unfulfilled and dissatisfied with life. The truth is that I was addicted to doing what had never been done. At the time, though, I wanted someone to blame for my dissatisfaction, and I chose my father.

Dad was not an especially good communicator, and he rarely talked about his feelings. Like many other people I know, I never heard my father say he loved me or offer much positive feedback. Most of the input I remember was in the form of criticism. For example, he didn't want me to have a steady girlfriend in high school or college because it could hinder my career. Now that I had a career, I didn't know what a healthy relationship looked like. I zeroed in on this and wrote him angry letters for his supposed deficiencies. He never answered them. This only confirmed to me that I was right. Even though a terrible gulf grew between us, I felt justified in my position. I had found someone other than myself to take the blame for the restlessness and emptiness in my life.

Blaming Dad didn't make my life any better. One night

I was telling my mother by phone how angry I was that my father would not admit any wrongdoing or responsibility for the neglect I felt I had suffered. She was quiet for a moment, and then she said, "You need to forgive him. You have hurt people, too, and you need to be forgiven."

This was the last thing I wanted to hear as a rising young neurosurgeon. Shouldn't he be apologizing to me and asking for my forgiveness? If I forgave Dad, then I would have to take responsibility for my own life and failed relationships. After I hung up the phone, though, her words stuck with me. I realized that I had hurt a lot of people and needed to be forgiven. The proper thing to do was to let my father off the hook and move on. That night in my bedroom I said out loud, perhaps to God, "Okay, I forgive my dad. I am responsible for my life, and I will stop blaming him." Nothing dramatic happened; I didn't even feel better immediately. Looking back, though, I believe that was one of the most critical decisions of my life. My choice to forgive slowly changed my heart, laid the groundwork for much of my future work, and soon opened the door to a major change in my career.

A few weeks later I received a call about a job opening in California. It was a clinical hospital position—not a position in which I would be teaching at an academic hospital. In the past I would have scoffed at such an offer, but something in my heart had changed. After forgiving my father, I found that the drive to be famous had ebbed away. I no longer felt that I had to prove myself to him or to my colleagues. So instead of dismissing the job, I considered it.

For some time I had wanted a better balance of work and leisure in my life. I wanted to be less consumed by work and have more of a social life. I dreamed of working in a place with a more temperate climate. My ambition had always bound me to a busy hospital, where prestigious careers were made. Now that fame was not my overriding goal, benefits such as good weather seemed much more attractive.

I made up my mind, and at thirty-two years of age, I took the biggest risk of my career up to that point, leaving a busy academic position in Pennsylvania and going to San Diego to work in a community hospital. My lifestyle changed instantly. Instead of working constantly in a stressful, cold-weather environment, I was now getting out to play volleyball on the beach. The natural beauty there was almost overwhelming. It had been a long time since I'd had time on my hands—now I had time to jog, time to think, time to consider my life.

I thought well of myself in those days and believed I was getting what I deserved out of life. I had worked my way up from a gas station attendant and had proved that people could achieve what they wanted if they worked hard enough. People who did not rise above their circumstances were weak, in my opinion. Deep in the recesses of my mind, I probably even believed I was somehow superior to the sick people whom I treated—thinking that if they had been exercising and taking care of themselves as I did, surely they wouldn't have such problems.

In my personal life, the material world remained powerfully alluring to me. I loved parties, concerts, and black-tie affairs. I dated often, and although I did not find love and contentment, I was doing my best to approximate them with adventure and escape. As for God, when I thought about him it was usually in a form such as this: *I have dedicated my life to serving others; I am doing God's work. Now, what should God be doing for me?* Obviously my life wasn't completely devoted to "others," and as for doing God's work, I hadn't sought God's opinion on how he might like the work to be done. But being in the business of saving lives, it was easy for me to assume I was doing God's work by default.

I had not given up my faith altogether. Rather, I free-lanced it, saying a prayer or reading the Bible when I felt like it in the privacy of my own home. I was careful not to let my faith affect my job or my social life.

Then one day I had a very strange conversation. Having just moved to San Diego, I was beginning to enjoy my new life there, which included jogging along the boardwalk on Saturday mornings. Somewhere deep inside, I knew that I was experiencing God's kindness. I believed that I deserved the blessings in my life, that I had made my own breaks; but my heart was more open to hearing the voice of God than it had been in years.

While I was jogging along the boardwalk one day looking for female pro volleyball players out practicing, a nonaudible, but nonetheless real, voice spoke to me: "What are you doing?"

I did not know at first if the voice represented my own thoughts or if God was confronting me personally. Either way, it seemed perfectly natural. I responded with the truth:

"I'm looking for women to date, as usual."

"How long have you been doing this?" the inner voice asked, with an emphasis on the word *long*.

I thought back to when I began to be interested in girls and did the math. "About eighteen years," I replied.

"What usually happens?" came the next question.

"Well, for the last few years, I meet them and then we spend about three months together. Then I get restless or bored and look for another relationship," I said inwardly.

"What do you have to show for all the time you have spent in pursuit of women?" the voice asked.

I had never considered this question. In all the thousands of hours I had given to my social life, I had never asked myself what was gained. I racked my memory for some redeeming result of all that time. I reached a dismal conclusion but delayed a little before answering.

"Nothing," I finally said. "I have nothing to show for it."

"Then how much time will you continue to waste?" asked the voice.

I said nothing.

"Why don't you stop looking?" the voice offered.

"But I'll die!" I said. "This *is* my life. I can't live without the hope of finding someone. It's the reason I get up in the morning. The hope of finding true love is my only motivation, outside my career."

The voice said nothing.

By this time I concluded that I must be having a conversation with God, since I would never come up with anything that sounded that crazy on my own. After some thought, I came to an inner resolution. "Okay, I will make you a deal," I said. "I will not approach any woman. But if a woman speaks to me, then I can ask her out on a date."

The inner voice did not object, seeming to concede this technical point to me. I jogged home feeling self-righteous and smart, knowing that I would still get plenty of dates. After all, I was a young neurosurgeon living on the beach in San Diego. Surely women would speak to me, or people would set me up on a date.

That's when the drought began.

One month went by without anyone approaching me. Then another. And another. I would stand behind women in the grocery store and bump into them, or help them with their carts, and still they wouldn't talk to me. I waited years, in the prime of my life, and not one woman I found attractive struck up a conversation with me; nobody set me up with anyone until several years later when I began dating again. It wasn't easy to stop pursuing women after eighteen years, but instead of being lonely, I channeled my energy in a different direction: getting to know God.

Soon after I made my "deal," I began to ask the question, What is God like? I took classes and began to study the Hebrew Scriptures, listening to lectures and reading the books of the Torah—Genesis, Exodus, Leviticus, Numbers, and Deuteronomy—for myself. I skipped over the genealogies but could not get enough of the wisdom contained in the stories. I alternated between these and the New Testament stories of

Jesus, also asking the question, Who is this? My appetite for wisdom grew, and soon I looked forward to taking time out of my schedule to read from the Bible. I would receive insights about my current circumstances and felt that God wanted to help me with his wisdom, which was far superior to my own. A new habit was forming, and after several weeks I truly enjoyed getting up early to spend the time in silence and solitude.

God came to a place of primacy in my life. As with any other relationship, the more time I spent with God, the more I got to know him—and not just as God the Father. Previously, my concept of Jesus had been that although he was a nice guy and loved children and the poor, he was unfortunately weak; it was his weakness that allowed the powerful people of his day to kill him. This is why I had been reluctant to follow Jesus before: I did not want to be weak, and I believed that Jesus had nothing of significance to say to a neurosurgeon like me who had the world at his disposal.

As I studied him now, I realized that Jesus had tremendous power, but what impressed me more was his restraint. He rarely used his power. I would have used that kind of power all the time, especially to heal people. I would have made myself a popular favorite as a healer—for the sake of healing but also in order that everyone would idolize and respect me. Just like the cure for cancer I wanted to discover—for the patients, of course, but also for myself. Jesus, on the other hand, was not trying to be famous or popular. He offended the people in control and broke their rules. I also saw something Jesus could do that I could not: love people who could do nothing for him. I generally cared for people when there was some benefit to me. I was nice to everyone, but Jesus actually saw value in everyone. I saw value primarily in the beautiful, the wealthy, and the intelligent. I would help the poor only as long as it was noticed by people I wanted to impress. I couldn't remember doing anything for someone less fortunate without telling people about it. Jesus' life shone a light on the gaping holes in my own.

Though I was going through a personal transformation, I still believed, stubbornly and arrogantly, that I didn't need a church. I liked my individual approach. I didn't see why church was necessary, at least for me. Playing volleyball or surfing was my "church." There was also another reason I avoided it: fear. I was still living in my identity as a Jewish doctor. I still attended synagogue. I wanted to have a private relationship with God without threatening my professional reputation or my social relationships.

Over the next several years, the curious desire to attend a church became stronger. It humbled me. Finally, I summoned my nerve one Sunday morning and drove to a nearby church. I sat in the parking lot, consumed with fear. *What if someone saw me? What would my colleagues say? What would the patients say who spoke to me as a Jewish doctor?* I had never corrected them. To build up my courage, I repeated to myself, "I am a free man. It's a free country. I will not live in fear of what others think—I am going in." Pushing my fears aside, I walked in and participated in my first Christian church service in twenty years.

I thought I had been free by not being chained to church, but in reality I had been living in a prison of fear of what others would think or say. Even my choice of churches was based in fear: I chose one with a pastor who was a Messianic Jew, who believed that Jesus was the Jewish Messiah. That way I could claim that the pastor was Jewish if any of my Jewish colleagues confronted me about it.

I began attending church regularly. The fellowship with others who followed Jesus became an important part of my life. One day the reaction I had feared from my colleagues came. A physician who had invited me over to his house for Jewish holidays in the past called me to his office. He was older than I was and had always been kind to me. I respected and enjoyed him and his family. We were chatting about a patient we shared when suddenly he interjected, "I understand you have changed your religion."

I was taken aback. He had obviously heard that I was attending church and was offended. There was an uncomfortable silence. I felt defensive, unsure what to say. This was the very situation I had been avoiding for twenty years.

I wish I had come up with something profound, even courageous. But like a scared schoolboy I blamed my mother.

"My mother is a Christian," I said, shrugging my shoulders, embarrassed and seeking to deflect the accusation.

"What do you think?" he asked.

I still wanted to be invited for holidays and feel loved in the Jewish community, but I couldn't betray my own conscience anymore. If I wanted freedom, I had to speak the truth.

"There is so much wisdom in the teachings of Jesus," I

said. "I have great respect and admiration for what he did and said, for the way he treated people."

I was stalling. We both knew I hadn't really answered his question. Then I found the courage of my father and continued, "I believe that Jesus is the Messiah." I stated it with a new conviction that I was speaking the truth and that it would cost me, as it had cost my father. In that moment I knew I had altered my relationship with that physician and with many other people in my life forever. He looked chagrined but did not say anything. His message to me was clear: this was not okay with him. Our meeting came to an awkward end.

It wasn't pretty, but somehow I had survived the kind of confrontation that had struck fear in my heart for decades. In the following months and years I was no longer invited to his home or to other Jewish homes on holidays, something I had long enjoyed. Of course, if my Jewish colleagues knew about my faith, it made no difference in our professional relationships within the hospital. On a personal level, though, some relationships turned distant. I felt the pain of these losses.

At the same time, I was experiencing the peace, energy, and freedom that come with integrity and authenticity. I had begun to break with past patterns of people pleasing and was learning to follow Jesus, who embodied authenticity and freedom. I was also learning that God has a purpose for every life—a purpose that may be vastly different and infinitely more worthwhile than the one we envision for ourselves.

CHAPTER 7

FORGIVENESS AS A CURE

WHEN I FIRST BEGAN PRAYING for patients, I had no idea that it would lead me to discover the power of forgiveness. The idea that bitterness was the source of health problems would not have made sense to me earlier in my career, but over time I became convinced that one of the greatest thieves of joy and health is the unwillingness to forgive the people who have hurt you.

I had confronted this lesson in my own life. After years of being critical, judgmental, and even envious of people I blamed for my shortcomings and failures, I came to realize that bitterness and envy were affecting my health and my enjoyment of life. When I forgave these people, I felt empowered to truly live. I became freer and happier, less driven to perform, less anxious, less insecure. As long as I held onto resentment, I felt compelled to achieve more and more in my field, mostly to prove that I was better than the people who had hurt me. The result was always dissatisfaction, no matter how much I succeeded in my professional life. When I forgave—beginning with my father but not stopping there—I ended this destructive cycle and began to change. It allowed me to see how to care for people in a new way, more selflessly than before.

I knew others needed to experience forgiveness as well, not just for psychological reasons but for psychosomatic ones. Emotions affect your immune system, for better or worse. Happiness heals like a medicine. Bitterness kills like a disease.[1] Releasing bitterness can dramatically help the underlying causes of many physical ailments, often more than any pill or procedure. I began to see harboring bitterness and resentment like smoking cigarettes: a lot of people smoke, but not every smoker gets lung cancer. Nevertheless, if you smoke, your doctor will ask you to stop. It is a deadly habit. In the same way I was convinced that resentment and bitterness caused some diseases outright and inhibited healing in others. I decided to bring it up with more patients and see what results I got.

I had no idea it would be so effective.

• • •

Ron was a tall, muscular man of about forty years, with cropped blond hair that suggested a military background. He worked for the U.S. Border Patrol, and he obviously lifted weights regularly. He wore a black T-shirt that revealed a massive chest and enormous arms, each the size of one of my legs.

Ron had a dangerous tangle of vessels in the dura mater, the covering of the brain. The technical term for his problem is dural arteriovenous fistula, or DAVF, which means there is a direct connection between the arteries and the veins in the brain. Normally, the two halves of the human circulatory system—the high-pressure arteries and the low-pressure veins—are kept apart by the much smaller capillaries. Capillaries act like transformers, stepping down pressure so that the arterial pressure doesn't overload the veins. Sometimes, for reasons nobody understands, rogue vessels form directly between arteries and veins, often in groups of twenty or more, creating a nest of high-pressure, thin-walled vessels that bleed easily. These high-pressure arterial vessels overload the thin-walled veins, causing them to dilate and become congested and engorged. This can lead to seizures, bleeding, and other problems.

DAVFs are a major headache for my patients and for me.

Ron's DAVF was causing him to hear the sound of rushing blood in his head, which was keeping him up at night. As he sat in my office, I explained his treatment options. Dural AVFs are complicated to fix because there are so many connections to block, and even getting into position to do the procedure can be difficult. He was quick to grasp everything I said and agreed with me that we should go forward with treatment. We scheduled the surgery for the next available date.

Before our appointment ended, I took the conversation in a different direction.

Ron had also complained of arthritis in his neck that was affecting his career and his enjoyment of life. He was unable to work because of neck pain and was out on disability. The arthritis was unrelated to his DAVF and is rare in people Ron's age. I could not explain why this young and physically active man had such debilitating disease in his neck. When things don't make sense to me, I begin to think about the possibility of emotional causes.

"Ron, there is something else I want to talk to you about," I said, clearing my throat and calling forth my boldness. "I want to make sure that you have every chance of healing from the surgery, and that means having good emotional health as well. Emotions can significantly affect the health of our bodies, for good or ill. Stress, anger, and resentment can have powerful negative effects on the body," I told him. "Bitterness is like an acid that eats its container."

He raised an eyebrow.

With my heart pounding, I looked this massive man in the eye. "Is there anyone you have not been able to forgive?" I asked.

He looked directly at me now, stunned. His eyes grew big and serious. An angry look passed over his face. He opened his lips, but no sound came out.

I was scared. It was the first time I had asked this, and it represented a new frontier beyond prayer alone. I was convinced that some health problems are spiritual and emotional in nature, but I didn't know which ones. Now I was testing the approach on a real, live patient—who happened to be about twice my size.

I studied Ron carefully. He had begun to puff up with emotion. It looked as if he was ready to launch out of the chair and come across the room at me. I scooted my rolling stool away from him, just to be safe, wondering why I was always pushing the limits and getting myself into new forms of trouble.

After a few long, painful seconds he deflated in his chair, dropped his head to his chest, and said something I didn't expect.

"My mother."

For a moment I thought I had misunderstood him. I was expecting him to say "father," or maybe "drill sergeant."

"Excuse me? I couldn't hear you," I said.

"My mother—I can't stand my mother. We haven't spoken in years," he repeated.

This man, who looked every inch the fearless marine that he was, had just acknowledged being poisoned inwardly by bitterness toward his mother.

"Do you want to tell me about it?" I asked.

Without hesitation, he began to talk, describing a sad tale of abuse and abandonment by a number of different people. Ron had felt rejected when his mother did not take his advice and chose instead to remain with a physically abusive boyfriend, a man who had hit Ron as well.

I was in new territory here, but I knew where I wanted to go next.

"I can understand your feelings," I said. "You have suffered injustice and you have every right to be angry. I do think that this is hurting your health and stealing much of the joy from your life. Bitterness is like poison that you swallow hoping that someone else dies. I am going to ask you to do something very courageous."

I paused for a few moments.

"I think you need to forgive," I said. "I don't want to push if you are not ready to let it go, but if you are ready, I would be happy to help."

He nodded.

"Yeah. What do I do?" he said.

"Do you have any religious background?"

"I was raised Baptist, but I left that long ago."

"Do you have any problems with my using the name of Jesus?"

"No."

"I like to use his name because he told us to forgive. He also loves to help us forgive, especially when it seems too difficult for us."

"Okay."

"Jesus made a very serious statement. He said that if we forgive others their offenses, God will forgive us. If we don't forgive others their offenses against us, God will not forgive our offenses."[2]

He looked genuinely surprised.

"I didn't know that," he said.

"I would like you to repeat a declaration of forgiveness.

Think about what I am saying. If you agree, say it as your own words."

"Okay."

I began to declare, "I choose to forgive my mother for the things she did and didn't do that hurt me. Specifically, I forgive her for . . . Now you continue. What do you want to forgive her for?"

Ron spoke. "I forgive her for making poor choices."

As soon as the words left his mouth, he began to weep. I got up and scrambled to find a box of tissues.

"I forgive her for thinking only of herself and not her kids," he continued. It was as if he'd been waiting to say it for years.

"I forgive her for drinking and not taking care of herself," he said with fresh tears, "and for rejecting me and choosing her boyfriend over me."

Ron went on to forgive his mother for not being there to support and help him when he needed her, and for emotionally and physically abandoning him. He was now crying so loudly that I hoped nobody in adjacent rooms or the waiting room could hear him. I handed him the whole box of tissues.

"Is there anything else you need to forgive her for?"

He thought a moment and wiped his eyes and nose.

"No, I think that's it."

"Would you like to ask God to forgive you for holding these feelings of resentment and bitterness against your mother?" I asked.

He was so ready that he didn't wait for my words but offered his own.

"God, please forgive me for holding this bitterness toward my mother," he said. It was as though a long silence between him and God had been broken. A sense of relief came over the room.

"If you have done anything that you would like forgiveness for," I said, "God would love to forgive you."

He nodded to affirm my words and asked God's forgiveness for some of his own failings.

"How can God forgive our sins?" I asked, drawing on Ron's church background.

"Jesus," he said simply.

"Would you like to thank him?" I asked.

"Thank you, Jesus," he said. "Thanks for paying for my sins."

We sat silently for a moment. I was still marveling at how the scene had played out.

"Very courageous," I said. "How do you feel?"

He dried his eyes and looked up with a big smile on his face.

"I feel like calling my mother," he said. "I can't wait to talk to her. Doc, I feel great, like a brand new man."

He hardly looked like the same individual who had walked in. His countenance had gone from stone to sunlight. There was a bounce in his step as we exited the exam room.

Three weeks later I operated on Ron. It was a difficult but successful procedure. It took six hours to plug up the large collection of arteries and veins that comprised the DAVF in his brain. Immediately after surgery he stopped hearing the annoying rushing sound, and we were both relieved. I saw him several times post-surgery, and he said his newfound joy was so strong that nothing could dampen it. He also said that the arthritis pain in his neck was so much better that he needed none of his pain medicine. He could hardly have been more different from the first time we'd met. He smiled constantly— it made me smile just to see him. His mother had recently turned her life around and had started attending church, and his family was planning a reunion. Much healing was taking place between her and previously estranged relatives.

This was my first experience with offering to help a patient forgive, and I have never seen a drug or an operation with that kind of transforming power. Forgiveness had turned a tough, angry, ex-marine into the portrait of childlike joy.

• • •

In the months after my first meeting with Ron, I took a number of patients through the steps of forgiveness for various offenses and situations. The results were amazing, each in its own way.

One man suffering from a small aneurysm and pain in his back and neck told me that he resented his real estate agent for getting him into a subprime mortgage right before the housing market collapsed. It was a situation that called for him to report the man to the authorities to prevent further harm to others, and he did so—but there were consequences for him as well: he lost his house and was living with his daughter. Also, his wife had died, and he was angry at God for taking his partner of forty-eight years. After releasing God from blame for the death of his wife and after forgiving his real estate agent for helping to get him into a financial mess, his attitude brightened, and to my surprise, his neck pain went away. Once he was talking with God, even though at first it was just to complain, he soon began to realize how God had blessed his life remarkably during those forty-eight years with his wife. This man—who had been given many treatments, tests, and scans and had spent many months looking for a solution to his neck pain problem—found relief when he released those he had not forgiven and was honest with God about the painful loss of his wife.

Another patient, a woman from a traditional Indian family, complained of daily, persistent headaches. She told me that she resented her twenty-one-year-old daughter for moving in with her boyfriend, a lifestyle that was very American but embarrassed their entire family. The daughter was now demanding money for school and expenses, though she was unwilling to live according to her parents' values. I suggested that my patient forgive her daughter for her choices and for demanding financial support. I also helped her separate her responsibilities to her daughter from her daughter's personal responsibilities. Her headaches went away immediately.

Rhoda, a woman in her forties, came in one day. She had a church background but hadn't attended in years. By now my presentation about forgiveness was succinct and fluid, and I told her how people's health can be affected by things in the past, especially things they can't forgive.

"It's interesting you say that," Rhoda said. "I was just telling someone last week that I think it's time I forgive my father. He's been dead for years, but he was such a mean man."

"You can begin the process today, if you would like. I'd love to help," I said.

She agreed, and I led her through the steps of forgiveness, as I had done with a dozen others by this time. She forgave her father for influencing her to marry an abusive man. She chose to set aside all questions of why God had allowed things to happen to her, focusing instead on the many blessings in her life that she had taken for granted. By the time we were done, a profound joy had come upon her.

"I feel light," she said, beaming. "I actually feel like going back to church and getting connected with God again."

"He has been waiting for you to set those things aside," I said.

"I'm so glad I did," she said. "I feel like he has rushed back into my life!"

She got up smiling and I walked her to the door, pleased that the conversation between her and God had been restarted.

Naturally, some people wanted nothing to do with forgiveness or "psychological" treatment. One well-dressed woman came in with a number of diseases: severe arthritis, thyroid disease, and sleep apnea, to name a few. She told me sarcastically that although she had seen many physicians, she got only two hours of sleep each night. I brought up the possibility that resentment or anger was affecting her—anger with God, with others, or with herself.

"I don't have any of those," she retorted.

I raised the possibility of her seeing a counselor but did not push the point. I moved on to talk about treating the possible medical causes. The rest of the visit went normally.

On a return visit to discuss a brain scan I had ordered, the first words out of her mouth were sharp and angry: "I did not appreciate your psychoanalyzing me the last time."

I swiveled in my chair to face her. "I'm sorry I offended you," I said. "That wasn't what I intended."

"I know," she said more gently, but her point was made. We talked about the artery in question, which the scan showed was not dangerous and not causing her pain. I didn't recommend any procedures.

She went on to ask if there was a doctor I could recommend for the puffiness under her eyes. It was clear she wanted to treat the symptoms, not look for the cause of her problems. I referred her to a physician who could possibly help, and she left my office. I never saw her again.

I don't bring up forgiveness with everyone, just those who seem open to it and in need of a greater remedy. Even for those who choose forgiveness, it is a process, not a once-and-for-all transaction. "Forgive and forget" does not usually work. It is a pursuit, a habit that takes time and effort, and the results are always worth it.

But sometimes overcoming the family situation and the

medical situation is extremely difficult—especially when the two collide.

• • •

Dave, a short, overweight man in his late forties, landed in the emergency room of the hospital one night. He had suffered a hemorrhage in his brain when an undiagnosed aneurysm had ruptured. Fortunately for him, the hemorrhage had been small and he was not actively bleeding.

I met him in the ER that night. In spite of the clear danger presented by his situation, his manner was blasé, defiant, distracted.

"How do you feel?" I asked.

"Little bit of a headache," he said.

I noted that his speech was clear, not slurred. The hemorrhage had bled into the cavities of the brain, but not its substance, and there was no damage as a result of the bleed. He had dodged a bullet.

"You're fortunate to have only a headache," I said. "Thirty percent of people don't make it to the hospital. When did this happen?"

"A few hours ago," he said.

"How did it happen?" I asked.

He was silent for a few moments, expressionless.

"I was fooling around with someone," he said. "I got a really bad headache all of a sudden. I knew something was wrong."

He didn't know it, but one of the most common times brain aneurysms bleed is during sexual activity. Many people don't exercise, so sex is the most stress their circulatory system experiences. Their aneurysm reveals itself at a very inconvenient time.

"Then what happened?" I asked.

"I fell down but was able to call my son," he said. That seemed difficult for him to admit. I sensed there was shame regarding the circumstances that had caused the bleed.

After reviewing the scans, I decided to do the surgery the next morning. Though there was a bleed into the brain spaces, called the subarachnoid spaces, there was minimal blood in the left temporal lobe where the aneurysm was located. If I had found an expanding blood clot, I would have rushed him into surgery, but there was not much swelling or pressure from the bleed. Dave was clearly awake and had not lost his mental or physical faculties.

In such situations there is no need to rush in, especially when the crew has just put in a full day of work. Doing technical procedures at night adds an extra layer of risk because the members of the team are not at their best; brains and bodies are clumsier when people are weary. The aneurysm had bled a little and stopped; Dave was not actively bleeding. There is a statistically small risk of rebleeding by waiting twelve to twenty-four hours with an untreated aneurysm. Because there is a statistically small risk of rebleeding and because these cases require significant concentration and technical skill, neurosurgeons typically wait until normal surgery hours to treat them.

"We're going to treat this first thing tomorrow morning," I said. "I need to discuss the risks with you. The aneurysm could bleed again during surgery; the procedure has a risk of stroke or death. Your problem is serious. Do you have any questions?"

"No," he said, shaking his head, his eyes avoiding my gaze. The headache was certainly bothering him, but it seemed there was more to it than that. He seemed numb to the gravity of his physical situation and embarrassed to have involved his son.

I understand that there is guilt and shame involved in many of the things that bring people to the hospital. It is like getting caught with your hand in the cookie jar. You have been doing your own thing over in the corner, and suddenly your little secret escapes. When some people get caught, they become humble and penitent. They recognize that they have gone too far and want someone to help them make peace with God and get rid of the guilt and shame. These powerful negative emotions can cause significant stress on our bodies. When we are in danger of facing consequences for our actions, the body responds with stress hormones that raise our blood pressure and keep us from sleeping as we think of ways to get out of our predicaments.

I didn't want to exploit the situation, but I wanted to offer Dave an opportunity to have a clear conscience if he had crossed a line somewhere. I sensed that he was feeling so ashamed that his health might suffer. I could have waited until the next morning, but considering even the small risk of his bleeding overnight, I felt that it was necessary to ask him now so that he could sleep. I lightly touched his forearm and looked at him with kindness.

"Were you raised with a faith or religion?" I asked.

"I was raised Protestant, but I'm nothing now," he said.

"This is a serious situation in your brain," I said in a soft voice. "If there is something you need to clear up or if you need to make peace with God, this would be a good time."

He looked at me with muted scorn, rolled his eyes, and exhaled sharply through his nose, mocking my offer.

"I would be glad to call a chaplain," I suggested, in case he was uncomfortable with his surgeon knowing the details of his life.

"No, I don't need that," he said.

Accepting this, I went on. "It is my habit to pray with patients. Your aneurysm has a risk of bleeding until we get it fixed tomorrow. Is it okay with you if I pray?" I asked.

While I waited, he looked around the room as if avoiding the question.

"I don't have to pray if you are uncomfortable," I said.

"No, it's fine," he said.

I put a hand on Dave's shoulder.

"God, you know all about Dave, and you love him. I am asking you to keep him safe tonight and to keep this aneurysm from bleeding until we can fix it tomorrow. I ask for skill and wisdom in surgery. In Jesus' name, Amen."

I left the ER, and Dave seemed as unconcerned about the aneurysm as when I first came in. His mind was on other things. I went home knowing I would see him again soon.

The phone woke me up early the next morning. Dave's aneurysm had bled again, producing a larger blood clot in the left hemisphere of the brain, where his speech and understanding centers were located. But since the left side of the brain controls the right side of the body (and vice versa), it was Dave's right side that was affected. When I went in to see him, his condition had significantly changed. He was having trouble speaking and understanding, and his right arm and the right side of his face were weakened, as if in the aftermath of a stroke.

There was another wrinkle: before we could get him into surgery, I was told by a nurse that the police were waiting to speak with me. Neurosurgeons are rarely surprised by any new twist, so I calmly walked into the waiting area to talk to them.

"Hello, officers," I said, shaking their hands. "How can I help you?"

"We're here to interview a patient of yours, David Jackson," one of them said. "We understand he was admitted last night."

"He was, but unfortunately he can't talk," I said. "The bleeding has put pressure on his speech center, and it's rather serious."

They paused, quietly frustrated.

"When do you think he might . . . regain his faculties?" one of them asked.

"There's a chance he may never regain them. We won't know for a week or so after the surgery, and that's assuming the surgery goes well."

They thanked me and left. I turned to the nurse, who had been hanging back, listening.

"I wonder what that was about," I said.

"I heard them say something about an underage girl," she said, then turned with disgust and went back to her duties.

I went into the room to see Dave, wondering about his life situation. He was no longer sitting up in bed, but lying back, his eyes registering alarm. He had not been informed about the police visit, but he seemed to know that his physical condition had gotten much worse in just a matter of hours.

"Good morning, Dave. How are you feeling?" I asked.

He tried to speak, but the words were unrecognizably slurred; the right side of his face was not working. He tried several more times to speak, but nothing intelligible came out. He exhaled hard through his nose and, with a look of frustration, stopped trying.

"That's okay," I said. "Can you move your arms for me?"

He moved his left arm, but his right arm remained immobile.

"Can you move your right arm?" I asked.

He moved his left arm only and smiled slightly as if that was what I had asked. When he smiled, I noticed that his face was not working on the right side. I held up his right arm for him and asked him to move it. Nothing.

"Do you know whose arm this is?" I asked.

He shook his head. "Ohh," he moaned, meaning no.

This new blood clot was putting pressure on the left hemisphere of his brain, causing something called spatial neglect, a condition that prevents a patient from feeling a limb or recognizing it as his own. He was becoming trapped in his own body, unable to move one side or to speak.

It was time to fix the aneurysm to prevent him from bleeding again, but this serious damage from the new bleed was something I could not fix. The techs were already preparing the procedure room, but I had an ominous sense that Dave's condition would continue to deteriorate. I also knew that there was something about his recent encounter that required the police to talk to him. I do not ordinarily bring up the issue after it has been rejected, but this time I wanted to give my patient another chance—perhaps his last chance—to get right with God.

I said, "You've suffered another hemorrhage, which is why you are having trouble speaking. This is an important moment for you. Is there anything you want to talk to God about? You can do it in your own heart without speaking any words."

He shook his head no. I gently grasped his hand.

"I'd like to say another prayer, if that is okay."

He shrugged his shoulders and stared straight ahead. I wasn't sure what he wanted, and I never want to push prayer on people who don't want it—even if they can't speak. So I asked again, "Is it okay if I pray for you? I don't have to if it makes you uncomfortable. I need you to nod your head if you want it."

He grabbed my hand and nodded his head. He seemed comforted as I spoke to God on his behalf.

Twenty minutes later I was in the reading room with my techs looking at the CT angiogram on the 3-D screen. There was Dave's aneurysm in all its three-dimensional glory. I spun the image around using the trackball to view it from all sides. This was a mean one, with multiple pear-shaped lobes and measuring more than ten millimeters, and he had a new blood clot that had not been there the night before.

Hemorrhages can repeat. Upon bursting, blood pours out of the aneurysm at high pressure (arterial blood pressure is normally 120 mm Hg), filling the low-pressure brain cavity (which is normally ten times lower, around 12 mm Hg). Dave's first hemorrhage had bled around the base of the brain, filling the cavities there but clotting off before doing any significant damage. The second hemorrhage had not clotted off as quickly, and the artery had shot blood up into the brain like a concentrated jet of water into soft mud. This had damaged centers of speech and mobility of his right side: face, arm, and leg. No wonder Dave was having trouble talking and moving.

There was really nothing medical science could do to repair the damage he'd suffered. We had to let the body take care of that. I was going after the aneurysm itself to prevent future ruptures.

I knew it was going to be tricky, and now I had a decision

to make: open surgery, by drilling open his skull and dealing with the aneurysm directly, or going through the vessel in his leg and closing the aneurysm off with tiny coils. Both options were worth considering. Open surgery would allow treatment of the aneurysm in person, so to speak, and this could arguably be more effective. I would be dealing with the actual vessel and would put a clip on it. There was something to be said for having that kind of access to a difficult aneurysm like this.

Still, an open surgical procedure would require manipulating Dave's brain, pushing its lobes apart to reach the aneurysm. That would cause more harm to his already injured left hemisphere and speech center. Damage is almost inevitable when you push a swollen, injured brain around on your way to an aneurysm. I concluded, as I watched the screen, that the best course was to do this with minimal invasion, leaving the damaged brain alone and going up through the vessels.

Moments later I entered the procedure room and saw Dave on the table, anesthetized and draped in blue cloth. I couldn't help but think of the visit from the police and Dave's defiance each time I had asked him about making peace with God. This wasn't just brain surgery; someone's soul was in the balance. My opinion was that Dave wasn't ready to meet his Maker. Maybe he felt as if he needed to suffer for his sins. Maybe he had a destructive lifestyle and wasn't ready to give it up. Whatever the case, something seemed unresolved.

I stood next to his body, inserted the needle into his

femoral artery, and got to work filling Dave's aneurysm with platinum coils. The tricky part would be filling the pear-shaped aneurysm in such a way as to inhibit the blood from reaching the dome of the aneurysm, which contained the rupture site. One coiled ball wouldn't do—that would leave room on the other side of the aneurysm for blood to flow around it. I would have to construct an effective barrier, essentially a small dike, or dam, to keep the pressure of the circulatory system from pushing against the weak side of the aneurysm. And I had to do it all within the tiniest of spaces.

I threaded the catheter up the left internal carotid artery to the base of Dave's brain. Through the main catheter I inserted a micro-catheter that had a guidewire with a curved tip. From three feet away I could rotate the wire and move it right or left, depending on where I wanted to go. Getting in was tricky, and I held my breath as I often do at this point, carefully advancing the micro-catheter over the wire and into the aneurysm.

Because in this procedure you are pushing from three feet away, the curvature of the vessels can absorb a lot of energy and mask what is really happening at the tip of the wire or catheter. If it builds up too much energy, it can jump forward. The last thing I wanted was the catheter jumping into the aneurysm and rupturing it. A significant number of people die or sustain permanent injury when an aneurysm ruptures during a procedure. Poke through a vessel or an aneurysm in the brain, and the brain cavity will fill with

blood—a dire emergency. It is one of the ever-present pos-
sibilities of every procedure I do.

With careful movements I avoided that outcome, and
within an hour, I was safely in position and ready for the detail
work. Into the back of the catheter I loaded my first coil, a
20-centimeter length of platinum wire that, when extruded
from a catheter, would form a 7-millimeter, three-dimensional
sphere. This would serve as the scaffolding. Slowly, with the
gentle force of my fingers, the first coil reached the aneurysm
and began to form its spherical shape. I saw it enter the aneurysm correctly and was pleased with the little "construction
project" so far. Although magnified on the screen, the entire
aneurysm was only about a quarter of an inch in diameter.

"Let's do a run," I said to my tech, and she changed
the working view on the machine to capture new images.
I stepped on the pedal to begin the digital subtraction angiography. The computer captured a picture of the skull and
brain with no contrast dye, then it signaled me to inject the
dye. As the dye coursed through the arteries, the computer
captured images at three frames per second and subtracted
out everything that was on the first picture of brain and
bone. That left a view of only the dye flowing through the
sharply delineated arteries and veins, without all the bones
to distort the view. It then played like a movie while I looked
for anything that didn't appear as it should. Was the coil
bulging into the main vessel? That could cause a clot and
a stroke. Was the coil poking through the back wall? That
could cause a bleed. Was there good flow into all the normal

vessels? I didn't want to damage one of them while trying to fix the aneurysm.

I love watching angiograms. I never get tired of seeing blood flow through the brain. The best is an angiogram of an aneurysm that bled but is no longer filling because the repair is perfect. That was the movie I wanted to see here, but I was only at the beginning. The moving picture of Dave's brain arteries popped up on the screen showing the aneurysm containing its new piece of "furniture"—the 7-millimeter coiled ball. It was perfectly placed.

"There we go," I said, as I slowed the movie down to watch it frame by frame.

The platinum ball was rather loose, and inside it I inserted another sphere, this one made of shorter wire and only five millimeters in width. The idea was to put progressively smaller coils inside one another, like Russian nesting dolls, creating a dense, hard ball that could resist the blood's pressure.

I inserted several more coils, checking each time to see what had moved in the process and whether the scaffolding was still in the correct place. Soon, I had a mass of metal coils filling one side of the aneurysm. Then I went to work on the other side, using a pair of smaller scaffolding coils and filling them with other coils until there was enough density to withstand the blood flow.

There was a time early in my career when I would have joked with the technologists about Dave's moral predicament, but not now. They didn't need to know any of his personal details to do their jobs. Dave was a person to me, not a mannequin. I wanted the best for everyone I worked on, and that meant leaving this man's private life as private as possible. During breaks in the surgery I occasionally prayed silently that God would give him another opportunity to live well.

Meanwhile, I was also performing the ever-present balancing act between using blood thinner and not doing so. Clots form on foreign bodies, such as the catheters and coils I was putting inside Dave's vessels. If a clot formed on the coils and was carried up the arteries into the brain, it could cause a stroke, making his debilitated condition even worse. The situation was complicated further by the fact that Dave's aneurysm had hemorrhaged—twice—putting his body on high alert for further bleeding. Injuries tend to make blood hypercoagulable (tending to coagulate more quickly than normal) to stop any further bleeding. This heightens the danger of a clot forming.

That was a strong argument for adding blood thinner early rather than later.

But how early? If I added it before the aneurysm was blocked off and, say, one of the coils poked through the wall, Dave would start bleeding and it would not stop easily.

I gave Dave blood thinner early because, in my experience, clotting is a more common problem than bleeding, but this made my task much more delicate. I didn't want to cause bleeding or clotting; each could result in Dave's not making it out of that room alive.

We were in surgery for two hours, filling Dave's aneurysm with coils. As usual, I wanted the patient off the table as soon as possible, but I also had to be extremely diligent and not rush through a single step. The last coils were the riskiest and most difficult. It is like filling the last bit of a bottle with water: it's easy to let it overflow. If the coil did not remain in the aneurysm, it would hang out into the artery and potentially cause another problem. If not enough coil was placed, the barrier would not be complete, allowing compaction of the coils and reopening of the aneurysm. It was tiring, focused work, but finally I had constructed a barrier I believed could withstand the relentless pulsing of blood.

"All done," I said, calling for the closure device that acted like a stitch in the femoral artery. Moments later I was outside the room reviewing the images from the case.

The angiogram showed that I had treated the aneurysm successfully, but everything looking good in the vessels doesn't mean the patient will wake up the same way he went to sleep. Because of the blood clot caused by the second hemorrhage, Dave's speech was still impaired when he woke up fifteen minutes later. In the recovery room after an hour or so, I checked his speech and the movement of all four extremities. Nothing had changed. I could do no more than let him recover and wonder again what sort of legal trouble he was in.

The next day while I was checking on Dave, I met Maureen. She had come in to get paperwork signed so he could receive a disability check. She said he was in danger of losing his apartment.

"How's he doing?" she asked with somewhat of an edge. She looked in terrible shape.

"You are his . . . wife?" I clarified before I gave her any information. She explained that although they had been separated for some time, they were legally married.

"We'll know more as he recovers, but the procedure went well," I informed her. "I am glad that you are able to help him with his disability paperwork. There is no way that he could do it."

It was painfully obvious that the situation had distressed her deeply. She seemed distraught, lost, casting about for answers.

"I can see you're stressed," I said. "This must be very hard on you."

She sighed heavily.

"It's a mess. It's a nightmare my kids have gotten dragged into."

"I'm not even sure what the situation is," I said.

"Oh, it's a wonderful situation," she said sarcastically. "He met a girl on the Internet who wasn't as old as she said she was."

That explains the police visit, I thought. She continued to talk freely, and I learned that Dave had suffered his burst aneurysm while this girl was at his apartment. By this time Dave had suspected that the girl was underage, and fearing that medical personnel would report him to the police, he called his son instead of an ambulance, and the son in turn called Maureen. While the son drove Dave to the hospital, Maureen tried to take the girl home, but she was a runaway. The girl began accusing Dave and even his son of rape. Both men were now facing legal charges.

Maureen was almost shaking with anger as she spoke.

"How are you dealing with it?" I asked.

"I'm not sure I am dealing with it," she said.

"Do you have family support?"

"Not enough," she said. "Our family has blown up. It's incredibly ugly."

"This may sound strange, but I think you're in danger in this situation too," I said, my head spinning a bit from the amount of drama involved.

"Tell me about it," she said.

"I don't mean what's happening with your family, even though that's obviously a problem," I said. "I mean you're in danger of having a lot of bitterness because of this. This is embarrassing for you and your family. You have every reason to be angry, even bitter—but that is not good for you."

She looked at me sideways, incredulous.

"*Bitterness* is a word I'm well acquainted with at this point," she said.

"In any case, it's a very powerful thing, and it can do significant damage emotionally and physically."

"What are you? A psychologist?" she asked, drawing the line I must walk with utmost care. I am a neurosurgeon, not a psychologist, and counseling is not my field or what my patients (or their families) expect from me. I am careful not to cross the professional bounds, and I offer to send many of my patients to psychological services for ongoing emotional and psychological care. Still, if I can open people's eyes to the power they have over the wellness of their own bodies simply by reconsidering their thoughts, I consider that part of my job.

"No," I said, "but I've seen a lot of people in bad situations get worse by holding grudges. It's not psychology, but I've seen a lot of people get better through forgiveness. If you want to talk more about it, you can come by my office at twelve thirty. I will have some time during lunch to chat."

Under normal circumstances she might have brushed off the offer, but she was like a drowning woman looking for a helping hand. Like many others I speak with in times of crisis, she was looking for someone who cared, someone who would give her knowledge and wisdom without judgment or ulterior motive.

Given the fast pace of typical health care, it is all too easy to move through a traumatic, life-or-death situation without having a chance to catch one's breath or think very far beyond the immediate present. I can fix an aneurysm, which has the benefit of extending life, but adding years to someone's life does not necessarily make it better. In many cases people's life choices are not working for them, and they have never considered that they can make different ones. A physician is perfectly positioned to be a healing balm, an advisor who tells people the truth in noncondemning ways, to appropriately help them sort out how they got to their present situation and where they could go from there. We occupy a place of trust in society, and we must honor that trust by sharing the best of our knowledge on how to treat our patients' problems, doing so with professionalism and respect for the patients' dignity.

She showed up to my office at twelve thirty sharp.

"Thank you for taking the time," she said as she sat down. She seemed more centered and in control than when we had first met.

"Let's take Dave's problems and set them aside for a moment so we can talk about you," I said. "The challenge you're facing right now is what to do with the pain and justifiable anger you have toward Dave. If you continue to rehearse all the offenses he has committed against you and your kids, the resentment will keep you awake at night."

She nodded.

"You have two choices: to hold onto it or to let it go," I said. "Forgiveness is a process, not a once-and-for-all transaction. Just as you probably made a habit of reviewing his offenses in the past, you will need to make a new habit of forgiving him from here forward."

She considered.

"I understand that. I guess I'm willing to try," she said.

"Do you think you can forgive Dave for this situation?" I asked.

"It would be pretty hard," she answered.

"That's fair," I said. "There is a lot to forgive, and you are in the middle of it now. Often people cannot forgive until things have settled down for a while. Even then, I think it may be the hardest thing that you will ever do. It is your Mount Everest. It will take courage and humility. If you aren't ready, I don't want to push you. You can take your time and come back when you are ready."

"I am willing to try. I still want the best for him. At least for my kids' sake," she said.

"Forgiveness is a process that we can start today," I said. "Again, it is not a once-and-for-all proposition. If you want to start letting go of the bitterness and becoming free, we can go through some declarations of forgiveness. I've seen this work for many others, and I'm sure it can work for you."

"All right," she said. "I'll give it a go."

One by one, with my leading, she named each of Dave's offenses and handed them over to God. It took about ten minutes and included things I often hear from divorced women: neglect, rudeness, lack of care and affection, out-right verbal abuse, abandonment, unfaithfulness.

"I cancel his debts," she concluded, repeating after me. "He owes me nothing."

When we were done, she looked up at me. "I feel better after that," she said. "I'm surprised."

"Let me mention something else," I said. "I'm going to guess that the problems in your marriage went both ways. It's pretty rare for one partner to be perfect. Usually there's some shared responsibility."

She nodded slowly.

"Yeah, I wasn't perfect," she said. "When I finally walked out, I left him with a lot of debt. I just hung it around his neck. That wasn't right."

"I bet you want to get rid of that guilt."

"I do, actually."

"Why don't you tell God and receive his forgiveness," I said.

"Now?" she asked. "Right here?"

"No pressure, but God promises that if we confess our sins he will forgive us and cleanse us.[3] I am thinking that you would like to get rid of that guilt and feel cleansed. You can do it privately if you like, but when you confess to someone else, there is more power to it, and people usually feel better.[4] Being honest about what you have done requires humility and courage, and God loves it when we demonstrate them by confessing. You can confess to someone you know and trust, or I would be happy to help you now," I said.

She nodded. "I'd like that."

"Tell God. I promise you, he is listening."

"Forgive me for what I did to Dave, knowing I was going to leave him," she said, and grabbed another tissue from the box on my desk to dab her eyes.

"When you said your marriage vows, did you promise to protect him and care for him?" I asked.

"Yeah, I think we said that," she sniffled.

"I understand the circumstances and Dave's behavior, but it sounds like you broke your promise," I said. "Did you make those vows before God and other witnesses?"

"Yes."

"God would love to forgive you for not keeping your marriage vows," I said without condemnation.

"Please forgive me for betraying Dave in what I did," she said, then turned to me. "But he betrayed me first."

"Then you can forgive Dave for betraying the vow that he made to you," I assured her, and she went on to do so.

Maureen paused for a moment before speaking again—and then it was as if the floodgates had been opened, and she was ready to deal with much more than just Dave's mistreatment of her. She talked about things that she had buried from her past but that had made her feel as if she didn't deserve anything good, anything beautiful.

When people share such things with me, it is a privilege to be part of the process, but it is God who does the work. After hearing her story, I asked, "Would you like to forgive those people and let it go?"

She closed her eyes and began to cry, silently at first, then with great heaves of her shoulders. After a while I encouraged her to express forgiveness in her own words.

"God, I forgive the person who made me feel like garbage for all these years," she said. "I'm done blaming you for not protecting me. I don't know why it happened to me or why this is happening to me now, but I'll take the chance that you're good. What else can I do?"

"You know, God sees you as precious and beautiful," I said. "I know you haven't felt that way, but it's good to speak the truth about yourself to replace the lies you've believed. Why don't you say, 'I am precious and beautiful'—that is what God says about you."

"I don't know if I can," she said. "I've never believed that."

I have suggested this a few times when it seemed to be what people needed to hear, because it is true—we are all precious to God—but they always balk at this suggestion. It is often so contrary to what they have believed for so long.

"You don't have to feel it, but when you say it, you're agreeing with what God says about you," I said. "It's not about giving you a good feeling, it's about agreeing with God."

"Then I am precious and beautiful," she said and broke down again.

"I'd love to hear you say it one more time," I said, and she smiled as she declared with more conviction, "I am beautiful."

As she repeated these words, her countenance began to change. The truth has that kind of power when we choose to engage it. So many people have been treated badly for so long that they begin to act as if they deserve that treatment. Maureen was rediscovering her God-given identity.

"Is that everything you want to clear up?" I asked after a moment.

"That's everything," she said. She looked up and wiped her eyes with tissue. She seemed fifteen years younger. Her face was no longer drawn. By all outward appearances she seemed transformed.

"I feel a tremendous peace," she said. "I feel really free."

"Good," I responded.

"I—I feel like I need more spiritual connection with God

in my life," she said. "I want to start going back to church. My boyfriend will go if I get him up in the morning."

"I think that's a great idea," I said. "You have been very courageous and honest today. I am really proud of you, and I know that God is as well. He wants you to get to know him. God is really amazingly good, and he is very patient and kind."

"I feel it," she said. She got up and hugged me, and I walked her out.

I saw Dave every day for the next week until he left the hospital. His speech remained slow, but the procedure had been a success. The coil barrier in the aneurysm held. Every day he consented when I asked to pray, but there was never any outward sign that he was open to God.

The police reported that the underage girl admitted that she had lied about having sex with Dave and with his son. Nothing Dave had done had violated the law—his headache had dropped him to the ground before he could go any further. In a strange way, his sudden aneurysm bleed had spared him a prison sentence. The case was dropped.

I saw Dave six months later. Speech therapy had helped him, but he still spoke slowly and not in complete sentences. His right arm remained weak, and it was clear that he would have a permanent deficit on that side of his body. This upset him because he wanted to go back to work but would be limited in what he could do. On the upside, the scans showed the coil construct was holding beautifully. I would not need to see him again for several years.

I thought he might be humbled by his recent dramatic

experiences and reconsider what he valued in life, including his own lifestyle and spiritual condition. When I asked him during his follow-up visits if anything was happening on his spiritual journey, he said no. He shrugged his shoulders and shook his head; he wanted nothing to do with it. His only concern was getting back to work and back to life as it had been before the hemorrhages.

I never saw Maureen again, but I felt confident that, unlike Dave, she had allowed the experience to open a new chapter in her life. Life is a continual journey. When people leave my office, I have no idea which direction they will choose to go. All I can do is to give them my best while they are in my care.

Early on, when I first began to pray with patients, God seemed to answer all my prayers and reward me and my patients with success. I began to think that perhaps I had found the key to perfect surgical outcomes. I even began to think that if I prayed, *I* could control the outcome and would never have a failed surgery again.

Boy, was that the wrong prognosis.

CHAPTER 8

PARALYZED

Sam was a thin man in his mid-forties, with straight black hair and a skeptical, serious personality. He was by most measures poor, having come from another country without a lot of advantages, but he was in the middle of a career change. He had returned to school to become a nursing assistant and had only a few more classes to take. He came to see me because he was having progressive difficulty walking and moving his arms. An MRI revealed the chilling truth: he had an intramedullary arteriovenous malformation—an AVM, which is similar to an AVF—in his spinal cord—that is, a thatch of abnormal and oversize vessels connecting an artery to a vein in the spine. As soon as I saw it, I drew my breath sharply and knew we were in for rough sailing. It was as if his body had created a problem designed to defy treatment.

Because the spine is part of the nervous system, the same system as the brain, neurosurgeons often work in this area as well. Spinal cord AVMs are the riskiest problems we deal with. Sam's problem had the additional disadvantage of being high up on the spinal cord, meaning that everything below his neck was at risk of being paralyzed if the surgery failed. To make matters worse—much worse—because the AVM had been forming for probably more than forty years, putting steady pressure on the vein, the wall of the vein had ballooned out and created a huge aneurysm in the middle of one of his vertebra. The aneurysm was one of the largest I had ever seen in the cervical spinal cord—two centimeters in diameter, so large that it had actually changed the shape of and enlarged the bony opening in his spinal canal. This naturally threatened the spinal cord itself, which was pressed against the bone by the aneurysm. The spinal cord was now compromised and was slowly being severed.

The spinal cord in a normal body is a rope of densely packed nerves about the width of your index finger, traveling down the neck and back. These nerves connect the brain with the body. Sam's spinal cord was no longer a thick rope but a thin layer of nerves draped around the aneurysm like a nightgown. All signals from his brain to his body were traveling through this ribbonlike connection. Any wrong move, any swelling, could irreparably damage the layer of nerves and break the connection, leaving him immobilized for the rest of his life.

Cases this risky showed up only every couple of years, and I soon realized that this would be one of the riskiest cases I had ever treated. There was no way to tackle it in a stepwise fashion, treating one problem and then waiting to fix the other. I couldn't close the AVM without closing the aneurysm, or vice versa. It was all or nothing. Both had to be treated simultaneously or not at all.

I explained all this to Sam. He understood that the spine was a dangerous area to be working in, but he stubbornly seemed to think that there was a way to treat it without real risk. Every time I told him what was at stake, he looked at me as if I were exaggerating or simply withholding the perfect treatment for his problem. Like some other patients, he had a hard time accepting that there were limits to modern medicine and that we had now reached the end of the dock, so to speak. What lay ahead were uncharted waters, but I explained that I would navigate them as best I could.

Unhappy with his options, Sam chose to delay treatment for three months and to continue in school. During that time he kept getting weaker. Walking became more difficult and he was losing dexterity in his hands, making his career goals impractical. All signs pointed to his being in a wheelchair in just a few years. Finally he called my office and told me he had decided to have surgery. No other option was available to him, and he was ready to take his chances.

I prepare extensively for each one of my cases, but

Sam's consumed me more than any other had up to that point. I started by going through the scans and asking myself the series of critical questions that I ask myself with every patient: What can be done? What should be done? How much can I do? Do I need to do it all? Is there any uncomplicated way to do this? Is there any way to postpone it and do it later? Where is the patient in life, career, and family? Should he or she be taking this risk now?

In this case the questions all led to the same conclusion: that Sam was better off trying to have this problem fixed now rather than waiting until it was too late. Perhaps we could salvage his mobility and give his body a chance to repair the damage in his spine that this malformation had quietly caused over the decades. Perhaps he would return to normal.

As I considered my options, I called a colleague to see if he had other ideas. He didn't. I spent hours thinking about the case and planning for the treatment. To close the aneurysm and the AVM would require that I inject glue to block the vessels comprising the AVM and plug the internal aneurysm—typical treatment for an AVM. How an aneurysm this large, and in an area this sensitive, would react was unknown. When the flow into the aneurysm was stopped and the pulsating blood was no longer expanding the aneurysm with every heartbeat, the pressure on the spinal cord could decrease. Alternatively, it might expand and put increased pressure on the spinal cord, causing paralysis. I prayed for God's wisdom and specific direction on this case that included so many variables. Ultimately, I was convinced that I had done everything I could to prepare, medically and spiritually.

I prayed with Sam in my office on his pre-operative visit the day before surgery. The next morning I entered the procedure room in my scrubs, donned a lead apron, and stood next to Sam, who was asleep from the anesthesia. The techs were busy prepping the instruments and the area on his leg where we would insert the hollow sheath and catheters.

One of the side benefits of praying with my patients is an increased emphasis on the personhood of the patient— I felt genuine concern for Sam, in addition to professional responsibility. At the same time, I am a specialized surgeon, and as I entered the operating room, I couldn't help but feel the thrill of taking on a "great case," the kind that is highly risky and especially difficult. Great cases give us the chance to test our skills against the toughest problems the body can come up with. They provide a challenge to be met.

The room was electric with anticipation and optimism. My heart was pounding. I was also keenly aware that it was Sam under that blue cloth, a man whose future was in my hands. The surgery was about him, not me, and I felt an overwhelming sense of responsibility to get it right.

The guide catheter went in quickly, up through the aortic arch and through a vertebral artery. Sam's vessels were surprisingly straight and flexible, probably due to his relatively young age and the fact that he was so thin. The micro-catheter also went into the feeding artery easily.

Within thirty minutes I had the micro-catheter in place in his spinal cord and was ready to do the injection.

Injecting glue into an AVM is tricky business. The glue that neurosurgeons use, a cyanoacrylate, is similar to super-glue, except that it costs $2,500 instead of $2.59. It even smells the same. When it comes in contact with blood, it hardens, sticking to itself and to the vessel wall and form-ing a blockage. The neuroendovascular surgeon mixes the glue in the operating room and makes the critical decisions about how thick it should be and how quickly to inject it. The thickness of the glue determines how quickly it will harden. If the mix is too thin, it will harden slowly and the glue can flow right through the desired area and into the veins, hardening there and causing the malformation to rupture. If the veins are large, the glue can travel to an unwanted place in the body, such as the lungs. If the glue is too thick, it will harden too quickly and block the feeding artery without going into the actual AVM. As a result, the AVM will continue to feed from smaller branches and you will have lost your access to it, making it harder to repair than before.

Before mixing the glue, I did an injection of contrast agent into Sam's AVM to measure how quickly blood flowed through it. The digital subtraction angiography, running at 4 frames per second, showed me how long it took for the blood to travel from the tip of the catheter in the feeding artery to the draining vein. This told me how much time the glue would spend inside the AVM before passing through and, therefore, how thick my glue mixture should be. His blood was moving quickly through the AVM.

Convinced now about what type of mixture I needed, I went to the back table and mixed the glue with metal powder and with the contrast agent to make the glue visible on the X-ray. I didn't dilute it much because Sam's blood was flowing so rapidly. I needed it to harden fairly quickly. I stirred the mixture in a small glass, then drew it into a syringe. I walked back to the operating table and handed the syringe to one of the techs, Lydia, who rocked it back and forth to keep the metal powder suspended until I was ready. I made a final practice run with contrast, and when I was ready, she handed the syringe to me.

Injecting glue is stressful. My technologists often have to remind me to breathe during those moments, because my whole being is focused on the shades of gray on the TV monitor that indicate where the glue is going. It is over in seconds and requires split-second decision making.

With a twist of my wrist, I attached the syringe to the clear hub of the micro-catheter, which was essentially now a three-foot-long flexible needle. I began to push the syringe plunger carefully, at just the speed I thought necessary. On the screen I saw the glue come out of the tip of the micro-catheter and enter the vessel. My adrenaline was flowing as I watched to see how the glue was going to respond once it hit the blood. Would it fly through the AVM and into the vein on the other side? Would it stop short of the AVM?

"Breathe," Lydia reminded me, and I exhaled.

I saw the glue flow, as expected, into the AVM and the aneurysm. Within seconds I could see it hardening.

"Come on," I said under my breath. "Stick in there."

The hardening glue began to close off the unwanted vessels and the aneurysm. The flow of blood narrowed and decreased. Soon, the flow was choked off entirely. I had put solid walls in the passageways of the rogue vessels. In a few brief moments, it was over, and I had done just what I wanted to do. Ninety percent of the problem had been closed in a single injection: the AVM had filled with glue and been almost completely shut down and the aneurysm was no longer filling. I felt as if I had just hit a triple in the World Series.

The case wasn't over yet, though. A small, peripheral area of the AVM was still filling with blood. I maneuvered a second micro-catheter into another artery that was supplying the AVM and did a second injection. The scan showed that this closed off an additional 5 percent of the malformation. Ninety-five percent of Sam's problem had been filled with glue in a matter of a few crucial seconds. It would be many years before the AVM would return and was unlikely ever to need treatment. Now it wasn't a triple, it was a game-winning home run.

I backed out the catheters before they became glued into the vessel, and I smiled beneath my mask, extremely pleased with the technical aspects of the case. I had judged the blood flow correctly, mixed the glue correctly, injected it at just the right rate. No normal vessels had been harmed, and the unwanted formations were cut off from blood flow. I was cautiously exultant.

Sam was wheeled into post-op, where we waited for him to wake up. It took longer than usual because the anesthesiologist had planned for a lengthier procedure than it turned out to be. I waited anxiously, exhausted by the preparation and by the adrenaline still circulating in my system. Half an hour later, in the recovery room, Sam stirred and I saw him moving his arms and legs. I came immediately to his bedside.

"Give my hand a squeeze with your right hand," I said. He did.

"Now your left hand," I said. He did that, too.

"Wiggle your toes for me," I said. He wiggled all ten of them. I had seldom seen anything more welcome or beautiful. Tears of gratitude and relief began to course down my cheeks. It was one of the few cases in my career that made me weep. The almost unbearable stress of the procedure drained away in an outflow of emotion. I grabbed his hand and said, "Thank you, God. We celebrate that you did what we asked of you. Now bless his recovery. In the name of Jesus, Amen."

I left the room and headed downstairs to prepare for the other case I had that day. I felt completely satisfied. Whatever doubts or fears I'd had were gone. We had passed through the fire and survived.

Then, in the midst of my preparations, I got a call from post-op recovery. Sam had stopped moving on his right side, and he was panicking. I rushed up as soon as I could. Sam's dark eyes were full of fear.

"What's happening to me?" he asked.

"Let's find out," I said. "Go ahead and move the fingers on your right hand for me." Nothing happened. A look of frustration and fear passed over his face.

"I'm trying," he said.

"That's fine," I responded. "Try the toes on your right foot."

Again, there was nothing.

"I can't make them work," he said. "Dr. Levy, I'm scared. What's happening? Why can't I move them?"

He was weak on his left side but flaccid on his right side. I turned to the nurse and ordered more steroids and other medications to decrease swelling, which I thought might be causing the aneurysm or veins to press against the tissue-thin spinal cord.

"I was fine," Sam said, his voice trembling with sadness and an undercurrent of anger. "When will I recover? What's going on with me?"

"I don't know, Sam," I said. "I'm doing what I can. Let's wait and see."

Our celebration had turned to uncertainty bordering on despair. I was watching someone who had emerged intact from a procedure slowly lose function, limb by limb. There was nothing I could do. In the next few hours I considered the different surgeries or options we might try to salvage our initial good result. I talked with my colleagues, searching for an answer I had yet to find, but they agreed that there was no solution that would not put him at more risk. We had done as much as we could to bring down the swelling. Now Sam would have to recover on his own.

I kept visiting him throughout the day, hoping and even expecting him to recover any time. Instead I watched all his limbs gradually lose their mobility as he grew more desperate and emotionally shell shocked. Paralysis was creeping over his body, stilling every movement, as the swelling pushed against the spinal cord and cut off the signals from his brain.

Within twenty-four hours, Sam was quadriplegic. He could move nothing below his neck. The worst outcome aside from death—some would say worse than death—had been realized.

Numbness came over me and I began to function automatically, my conscious mind unable to process the grief. I rarely suffered such an emotional blow from a failed procedure, but I did not have the luxury of taking time away to recover. I had a terrified patient and his angry, frightened family to deal with. My emotions had to be set aside so that I could make important decisions and walk them through this tragedy. I also had another case to do that day and could not be distracted by thoughts about Sam.

I visited with Sam the next several days. We prayed every time, along with his sisters who were there, that God would reverse this paralysis. *Maybe the swelling will ease and the spinal cord be restored*, I thought. Maybe he would regain mobility just as unexpectedly as he had lost it. Every day he asked me, "Dr. Levy, when am I going to get better? When will I be able to walk?" Every day that went by without his recovering normal function meant a greater chance that his paralysis would be permanent.

With some of his chest muscles now paralyzed, Sam developed a serious case of pneumonia. As I watched him suffer in these multiple ways, I was overwhelmed by my own sense of failure, even though I still believed that I had done the surgery almost perfectly. Doubts and fears tore at my confidence like jackals. How could this have happened? Was I losing my touch? Had I used the wrong glue mixture? Did I get enough counsel from others? Should I have done the procedure at all?

Deep inside, I also felt betrayed. Wasn't prayer supposed to prevent such things? Hadn't Sam and I petitioned God for a good outcome? Hadn't I even asked for prayer from people at my church for this case—something I had never done before? Hadn't I spent hours planning and asking God for wisdom? How could God let this happen? How could God treat this man this way? This was a motivated man who was going to school to train for better work. Of all my patients, why this one? A sense of devastation and loss overshadowed my every waking moment, and nothing would stave it off.

As I continued to visit Sam to monitor and pray with him, it was clear that the outcome was ruining him emotionally. He was distraught and desperate, inconsolable, constantly asking what could be done to restore the use of his arms and legs. It occurred to me that perhaps the pneumonia he had developed after surgery would keep getting worse and he would die, sparing him what he dreaded: life as a quadriplegic. Perhaps that was the only bearable outcome for him. Maybe it was God's severe mercy in this situation. Instead, his pneumonia improved on antibiotics, and it became clear that he would live—but his life would be radically changed.

I could have used a month off to recover from the case, but the following week I had other surgeries scheduled. I had never cancelled a case because of a bad outcome on a different one, and I did not want to start now. In truth, I did not even have the strength to call a patient to cancel. I was mad at God. I had trusted him and he had let me down. I began to wonder if I could even operate again. Or was I just scared that God had left me or, worse, had never been with me and it had all been my imagination? When it came to the big stuff, a high-risk case, God had abandoned me. I felt utterly alone.

My next operative day was one week after Sam's surgery, and I wasn't looking forward to it. With Sam lying in a bed as a quadriplegic at the other end of the hospital, I ascended the stairs to the pre-op area. This time I felt mechanical and joyless. I saw nothing good in the circumstances, but neurosurgeons are trained to lock their feelings away and operate on willpower alone. I had been trained to handle tragedy with poise and calm, never showing fear or self-doubt. Sam was my first major disaster since I had begun praying with patients. Commonly among surgeons, all previous successes are forgotten in the face of tragedy. In "autopilot" mode, I smiled at the nurses and pretended nothing was wrong.

Robotically, I checked the chart and reviewed the documentation for the procedure. Any warmth I gave off was manufactured; inside I felt as cold as the clamps and scalpels on the operating table.

Then came the moment when I had to approach my first patient since Sam, which meant offering prayer. I hesitated. Here was a hurdle too high. Would I pray with the patient waiting for me behind the pre-op curtain? How could I? I felt no connection to God; I didn't even feel connected to myself anymore. I felt remote, abandoned. As I searched my soul in that moment, I felt well justified in not ever praying for another patient. Why would I, when the results were so random?

Who was God not to answer my prayer for Sam? Surely, of all the prayers I had offered, this one should have been at the top of the list. He had answered prayers for many other patients who seemed, in my limited understanding, less deserving. But this time prayer had not helped, and instead of being the hero, I was the instrument of destruction. Had I not operated, he would not have been paralyzed, at least not immediately. Was this how I was rewarded for taking the risk of praying with patients? I had made myself vulnerable to them and to God, and God paid me back with failure? *No thank you*, I thought. *I'll take the conventional, safe route and hide again behind the facade of perfection, the illusion of control, retreating to safety from emotional involvement.* I would be friendly but aloof and distant once more. In my pain and frustration with Sam's case, I began to doubt God's care.

Of course other surgeries had involved complications, and some had even gone poorly or failed to solve the problem, but I hadn't experienced anything as wrenching as this since I began bringing prayer into my practice. Prayer had raised my expectations, and now I felt betrayed. Was God listening if I couldn't feel him? What would be the harm of not praying today?

Just as my thoughts reached a crescendo of confusion, a simple phrase came forcefully to mind: "Do the right thing." I recognized those words. I had heard them when I first began praying for patients and feared what others would think of me. They now gave me a new and unexpected sense of resolve. The phrase swept away other arguments like pieces removed from a chessboard. The answer was obvious: the right thing was to go against my feelings and do what was good for the patient. I had seen the results and could not deny that praying was the right thing to do, even if in my anger I didn't feel like it was. I hesitated no longer and walked up to Lupe, a fifty-seven-year-old grandmother with a brain aneurysm, and smiled as best I could. She had no idea what my last week had been like. With some emotional difficulty, I reviewed the risks of death, blindness, paralysis, and coma that could result from surgery in the vessels of the brain. Each word haunted me, as images of Sam lying immobile in his bed flashed through my mind. Lupe said she understood the risks.

"Do you really?" I wanted to say.

Instead, I spoke the words that by now had become

routine to me: "It is my habit to pray before surgery. Would that be okay?"

"Yes," Lupe said quite willingly. I had never prayed for a patient while suspecting that God was not interested in helping me or the one with whom I was praying. I didn't know if I would be able to go through with the prayer or if I would stop in the middle and not be able to finish. I put my hand on her shoulder. Out of sheer habit I began, "God, thank you for Mrs. Cortes."

Somehow as I said the words, I began to feel again—the ice around my heart began to melt. The more I prayed, the more energy I received; the fog lifted. I continued to my conclusion: "I ask for wisdom and success for the surgery. In Jesus' name, Amen."

It was not a long prayer, but by the time I finished, I felt something that had been missing for days: hope. I had begun the prayer purely out of conviction that it was the right thing to do, but I had ended it knowing that my doubts had been misplaced. God was at work and I did not want to operate without him, even if I didn't get what I wanted. The pain had caused the fire in my heart to go out, but he had blown gently on the embers hidden deep in the ashes.

Lupe smiled. "Thank you," she said. Then something happened that had never happened before. From the other side of the curtain separating one gurney from another, I heard a deep voice say, "Hey, Doc, when you're finished there, would you come over here and pray for me? My doctor didn't pray with me."

Lupe and I smiled, and I felt tears form in my eyes. God had not abandoned me. He was here with me as I did my best to care for the people that he sent my way. I walked around the curtain and found a man who was alone. His name was Travis, and he was the pastor of a church. He was having abdominal surgery that morning, but for some reason his wife and family could not be there with him, and he was afraid. I put my hand on his shoulder and reminded him that God was with him as I prayed for his surgery. When I opened my eyes, he was crying and wiping his eyes. He heaved a sigh that was so loud it might have summoned the nurses to see what was going on. He smiled at me, relaxed and at peace. I smiled too, patted his shoulder, and walked out of the pre-op area.

As I walked down the hall, I felt at peace, too, as if God were telling me, "I haven't abandoned you. Remember, it's not about you. There is no formula for getting your way, and pouting only shows your immaturity. Trust me with what you don't understand. I love you very much and nothing can change that. My love for Sam is greater than yours. I invite you to ask me for whatever you want, but prayer does not guarantee the result."

Lupe's surgery went well, and she went home the following day. As for me, I had found my way through a major crisis of faith. Doing the right thing when I didn't feel like it had brought a blessing to two patients, Lupe and Travis. I had chosen to trust the character of God and not my feelings. He was good even when I couldn't see it.

But there was still Sam.

• • •

Sam stayed in the hospital three weeks before being released and sent to a nursing home. He had not regained his mobility. Three months later he and his sister came to see me in my office. I cringed when I saw his name on the schedule. He was the last person I wanted to meet with. Seeing him would dredge up all the feelings of failure, betrayal, and personal grief at his incalculable loss. I had seen the wheelchair being pushed past my office door and could already feel the disappointment. Before going into the exam room where he was, I took a moment alone in the bathroom; splashed some water on my face; and prayed, "God, help me."

I paused outside the exam room door. It took all the strength I had to finally walk in. I knew it would be difficult to see him, and it was. He was in a wheelchair, emaciated, completely different from the man I had first met. He had recovered a little movement of his left arm and leg, but his right side was spastic and stiff. He had learned to use some prosthetic attachments to feed himself with his left arm, but both hands had fingers like claws with wasted muscles. I sat in my chair and looked at him. "How are you, Sam?" I asked.

He didn't answer but made a gesture with his head that was the equivalent of, "What do you think?"

"Tell me about the surgery," he said bluntly. "What went wrong?"

I slid my chair over to the whiteboard, where once again I drew pictures of his spine, aneurysm, and AVM. I explained in as much detail as I could what might have gone wrong—the precarious aneurysm, and the lack of tolerance for swelling of any kind—hoping that he would be satisfied and find peace with the outcome.

"Sam, I never wanted this for you," I said as I finished. He looked away. "I can't tell you how sorry I am that this happened," I said.

He said nothing.

I offered to say another prayer; I had nothing else to offer him. It seemed trite considering the many that we had already said. He nodded unenthusiastically. He was wearing a sweat-shirt, and as I put my hand on his shoulder, I realized just how much he had wasted away. There was hardly any muscle; it was all bone. I said a prayer asking that he would walk again.

I opened my eyes. Sam had never closed his. He was staring at the far wall, smoldering. A few minutes later, after we had gone through the necessary information for his checkup, his sister wheeled him out of the room, and I left it, too, as if walking away from a problem too difficult to face.

I didn't see Sam until a year later, when he returned for another checkup. An MRI showed that his spinal cord had changed completely. It was small and withered below the damaged area, and he had developed a severe bend in the angle of his neck.

When I had finished talking to him about his latest developments, he looked at me with pain-saturated eyes.

"What happened?" he asked again. "Why did the surgery leave me like this?"

"Sam, we've talked this through many times," I said. "I am very sorry that this happened to you. Yours is the case that has bothered me more than any other in my career."

He did not appear comforted, and I could tell that he was angry with me.

"Is there anyone who can help me?" he asked.

I wrote down the name of a doctor who specialized in scoliosis, but I knew that more surgery would not help him. He was grasping for solutions that did not exist. I prayed for him again before he left, but he remained as upset as he had been a year earlier. The prayer made me feel better but seemed to do nothing for him. His body had not healed, and neither had his spirit.

No surgeon likes to deal with complications, poor outcomes, or unhappy patients, but time generally allows us to let go of past cases. Sam's stayed on my mind. Three years later, I had a nagging feeling that I needed to see him one more time. I wasn't sure why, but something felt unfinished. I wanted to see again how he was doing before he slipped away into my past. I could have asked him to come in and see me, but I knew what was required for someone with limited use of his arms and legs to get to the hospital. My only other option was to go visit him. Though calling a former patient is not necessarily unusual in the course of follow-up care, asking to visit one is out of the ordinary for me. Yet I felt that I needed to make this exception. I called him one afternoon from my office.

"Sam, it's Dr. Levy," I said. He paused for a moment, clearly surprised.

"Hello, Dr. Levy," he said. I continued on quickly so he would not think I had come up with a new strategy for restoring his mobility.

"I don't have anything new to tell you, but I was wondering if I might come by and visit you sometime when I'm in that part of town, just to see how things are going."

It seemed as though he didn't know what to say at first.

"Fine," he said warily. "Sure. I don't mind."

"Great. I'll call you in advance," I said. "I hope it will be in the next few weeks. I'll see you soon."

"Okay," he said.

A few Saturdays later I drove to his neighborhood and parked my car in front of the small home where he now lived with his mother and sister. His sister answered my knock on the door and invited me in. Sam was there in his electric wheelchair. He gave a weak smile when he saw me, a little surprised that I had followed through on my promise. He was dressed in sweatpants and a sweatshirt; he looked gaunt like a rag doll, and miserable. His black hair had lost its luster, his brow was furrowed, and his face was joyless. He could move his left arm just enough to run the chair by way of a joystick. His right arm was rigid; he was unable to move it in any useful way.

I sat on the couch opposite him and struck up a conversation.

"So tell me what you've been doing," I said.

"Not much," he said with little attempt to appear happy. He let several seconds lapse between phrases. "I get outside occasionally. I found some alternative therapies on the Internet."

"Oh? What kind?" I asked, hoping that he had finally found a reason, any reason, to hope.

"Aromatherapy," he said. "But it doesn't actually help. I mean, what can help me now?"

With his chin he indicated his own skinny body in the wheelchair. Though he said nothing after this, I felt again that he was seething with anger toward me. I had felt this before from him but had forgotten about it in the months since we'd last met. It felt harsh and accusatory. He was staring away from me in silence.

I had come only with the intention of making a friendly visit, seeing where and how he lived and sharing a bit of his life, perhaps even "growing" from the experience. Now, however, I sensed that I needed to do something else: apologize to him. This was not something I had ever done to a patient before, and I didn't like the idea. After all, I had done my professional best on his procedure. Using my skills, I had even given him a chance at a normal life, when other physicians might not even have tried. I had already told him many times how sorry I was that this had happened, even telling him at one point, "We prayed about it, and still it happened," hoping that he would stop blaming me and take up the matter with God. Something still told me I needed to apologize for my part in putting him in the wheelchair. I had done my best, but that did not erase the fact that he had trusted me and I had injured him.

I felt uncomfortable with the idea because I knew it was not required of me, yet I felt impressed that Sam needed something from me so that he could move on. I sat on that couch and wrestled inwardly, not sure that I could do this even if I wanted to. My pride resisted, but my compassion pushed me on. Finally, after a long, tense silence, I decided that whether or not I felt I was in the right, I was willing to humble myself if it might help him to heal. I knew from my study of forgiveness that an apology is the most helpful step in opening someone's heart and encouraging him or her to forgive. I cleared my throat.

"Sam, I am very sorry for what happened to you," I said, using the same words I had used in my office a number of times. "I never meant for it to happen, and it is the last thing that I hoped would happen. Your case is one of the most painful of my career."

It was the quintessential professional apology, conveying how bad I felt about his condition without accepting any blame. He nodded and looked into empty space. He had heard all this before. Although I could justify myself in a court of law, we were not in a courtroom. In order for him to heal, I needed to apologize for my part in his pain, and it would be one of the hardest things I had ever done. Taking an enormous risk, I continued, slowly and deliberately.

"Sam, I want to apologize to you for what happened. The procedure that I did paralyzed you. You trusted me, and I let you down."

He turned to me with a startled look in his eyes, as if asking me silently, "Did you really say that? Did you really mean it?" Then, as if I had uncorked something inside him, tears began forming in his eyes faster than he could wipe them away with the back of his clumsy, partially paralyzed left hand.

"Lorna," he said, calling his sister. Then again sharply, "Lorna!"

I froze. What was happening? Was he angry? Was he going to do something radical, perhaps call the police?

"Bring me a tissue."

Lorna came in with the box and dabbed her brother's eyes. Sam nodded for me to continue.

"I don't want to pressure you to forgive me if you are not ready," I said. "This is not about my trying to feel good; it is about your becoming free. If you have resentment, anger, or bitterness toward me, it is not good for you or for your health. I want you to be free from it so that you can heal."

I waited for his answer while a battle raged inside my head. I was used to helping people get rid of their resentment toward others, but never against myself. I felt exposed and undefended. Then the old doubts about the surgery flooded back with their original force. Had I used the right mixture of glue? Had I been trying to be a hero, to show other doctors what I could do? This patient suffered daily while I continued to enjoy my life. Maybe I was just doing this to assuage my own guilt. I certainly had not come for this purpose, but I stood to benefit emotionally if he would forgive me. Would I be misunderstood? Were my motives pure? Had I ever had a pure motive? As uncomfortable and dangerous as it was,

I wanted him to be free from his bitterness. I wanted him to heal in every way possible.

Sam was still crying.

"Maybe we can walk through the steps of forgiveness together," I said. "Would you like to do that?"

He cleared his throat, nodded, and said, "Yes."

"Then repeat after me," I said, beginning with, "I choose to forgive Dr. Levy . . . ,"

"I choose to forgive Dr. Levy . . . ," he said,

". . . for the things that he did, . . ."

". . . for the things that he did, . . ."

". . . that hurt me."

". . . that hurt me."

"Specifically, I forgive him for . . ."

"Specifically, I forgive him for . . ."

"Now, what do you want to forgive me for?" I said, indicating that he should now say specifically what he was forgiving. He hesitated. *God, don't make me put these words in his mouth*, I thought. *It's too much.* Yet he said nothing. He would not move forward unless I led him.

After an awkward moment I finally said, ". . . for putting me in this wheelchair." It hadn't been my fault, but Sam had been holding it against me, since there was no one else for him to blame for the tragedy, and I needed to humble myself and allow him to release his bitterness.

". . . for putting me in this wheelchair," he repeated as the dam burst and he began to cry again.

"I forgive him for what my life has been like since the

surgery," I said. Tears now filled my own eyes as he repeated the words. *God, can I do this?* I wondered.

"I forgive him," I said, my voice cracking as I choked back my own tears, "that I can't walk." He repeated it as I grabbed a tissue and wiped my eyes.

"I forgive him for all the things that I have not been able to do since the surgery," I said, and he repeated it. It was taking real effort now for me to get the words out without breaking down.

"I set him free," I said, but he did not repeat it.

I looked up at him. I realized in that moment that I did want to be free of his anger. But Sam did not repeat those words. Instead he said, "I set myself free."

I smiled and felt peace fill the room. Though I had offered Sam the opportunity to set me free from his blame, his forgiveness had set himself free from the need to blame at all.

"Yes," I said, agreeing with him, "I set myself free from all anger, resentment, and bitterness." He repeated this after me.

"And I am confident that God will treat Dr. Levy," I said, swallowing hard as I continued leading Sam, "according to his justice . . ."

I said this with great trepidation. He repeated the phrase.

". . . and mercy," I concluded.

". . . and mercy," he said.

I paused for a moment.

"How do you feel?" I asked.

"Better," he said, smiling. The tears had stopped, and he was beaming in spite of himself.

"When we forgive others their offenses, God wants to forgive us.[1] You have forgiven me, and now God would love to forgive you for anything and everything. He sent Jesus to pay for your sins so that you can go free. Would you like to have your sins forgiven?" I said.

"Yes," he responded. With my leading he prayed, "God, please forgive me for my resentment and bitterness. Because you want me to forgive people . . . and until today I had not."

When he had finished, he looked directly at me for the first time since the surgery, no longer angry but appreciative.

"How do you feel now?" I asked.

"Much better," he said with the biggest smile I had ever seen him wear. He looked like a different person. The minute-by-minute misery he had previously embodied was gone. Now his smile was genuine. He was healing on the inside.

I asked if I could pray for his physical condition again, and he agreed. After I said "Amen," he looked at me.

"I feel an electrical sensation going down my spine," he said softly. "And . . . my right leg is moving better."

In the next few weeks, Sam found a new physical therapy program—and new strength. Within six months he was able to support himself with his arms and walk between parallel bars with the help of a therapist. He called to tell me, his voice exuberant, childlike, full of hope.

Sam and I both hope that someday he will walk again unassisted. Whether or not he does, the day that he forgave me was the day he released himself from his prison.

CHAPTER 9

THE GIRL AT THE BRINK OF DEATH

AT TWO YEARS OLD, Annette was one of my youngest patients, but I couldn't have been more impressed with her personality. Though most kids are afraid of doctors, Annette trusted me implicitly and came without fear when I asked to examine her. She was well mannered and remarkably sensitive to those around her. If someone in the room sneezed, she would say, "Bless you." She seemed tuned in to the needs of others in a way I didn't know was possible for a child her age. Never aggressive, she was actually a bit cautious. When she approached an unevenness in the pavement or a small downward step, she would turn around and slowly ease herself down backward. She was loving and polite, a joy to be around.

Annette's parents brought her to me because she had a quarter-sized pulsating bump on the back of her head, behind her right ear. It appeared to be causing her discomfort. She was not sleeping well, and she touched the area as if it bothered her.

In the exam room I felt the pulsating region, and though I had no confirming evidence yet, I was pretty sure that the angiogram would show an aneurysm that was only a small part of a larger DAVF (Dural Arteriovenous Fistula). When I did the angiogram, not only was there a DAVF, but it was surprisingly large for a child her age. It was a massive nest of connections between arteries and veins, and those veins were overloaded from the high arterial pressure: there were many dilated connections between the arteries and veins, and the improper connections were causing the formation of a large arterial aneurysm that we could feel through Annette's skin, though the largest part of the DAVF was inside the skull.

It was obvious we would have to do something, but all the possible complications of operating on such a young child sprang to mind. The amount of contrast dye you can use in children is limited because it can be toxic to the kidneys; this means you have to be judicious with it and work with images of lesser quality. The blood volume in children is very small, so blood loss is much more serious and could necessitate a transfusion sooner. Also, their body temperature can drop quickly—they don't have the body fat to keep them warm and intravenous fluids cool the body—so we have to keep children under heating blankets and warm the fluids we use.

More important, closing off the DAVF would require a long and involved procedure with lots of radiation. I did not want to expose a two-year-old to that much radiation if the DAVF was not posing an immediate danger. Since her only symptoms were apparently being caused by the aneurysm behind her ear, after some consideration I decided to recommend gluing that aneurysm shut and leaving the DAVF in her brain alone until later. The older she was, and the longer we could wait to repair it, the better for Annette. Her parents agreed with this approach.

I performed the procedure. The gluing of the aneurysm went well, and Annette went home the next day. She came back to see me two weeks later, and the mass was no longer pulsating. She was not complaining of any pain. I was pleased, as were her parents, and I happily escorted them out and made an appointment to see Annette again in a year.

Three months later they were back in my office. Once again Annette was not sleeping well, and she was blinking her eyes strangely. The area I had glued behind her ear was still not pulsating, but it had now more than doubled in size and was engorged with blood. DAVFs can grow by recruiting nearby arteries, and this one appeared to be changing. I told the parents that, by the looks of it, the temporary measures had not worked, and it appeared we would need to shut down the DAVF by trying to close the large vein draining the right side of the brain. This would leave only the vein on the left side to drain the brain of blood. Since that vein was large and healthy, it could handle the extra flow. Still, I could not predict how the brain of such a young child would respond to having a large, draining vein closed. This would be a major procedure with higher risks than before, but we did not appear to have any choice. She was getting worse.

Annette's parents were not particularly religious, although they attended church occasionally. They considered my words carefully. The mother was pregnant with twins, and I thought perhaps this was complicating their decision.

"We can wait until after your delivery to do the procedure," I suggested. She just smiled.

"I'll have plenty on my hands after they're born," she said. "I'd rather try to take care of Annette's problem now."

The father nodded and said, "I agree." With their decision made, I began planning for the procedure.

I spent much time studying the previous scans and plotting out the potential paths I could take to the DAVF in the back of Annette's head. Finally, the day arrived, and I walked in to see Annette's parents and both sets of grandparents in the pre-op area. Annette was in a crib, playing with a few toys. She looked up at me and smiled guilelessly, not knowing that soon we would be together again in an operating room, with her unconscious and me manipulating tools in her skull. I went through my usual recap, reminding the family of the risks and what we wanted to accomplish that day. At the end of the talk I said, "I'd like to pray for Annette."

Everyone circled up around the crib, surrounding Annette with love. She looked at us curiously.

"Father God, we come to you asking for success in this procedure today," I said. "I pray for wisdom and skill in my work. Give this family your peace. In Jesus' name, Amen."

We squeezed each other's hands; Annette smiled and continued playing with her toys. I left pre-op, and thirty minutes later joined my crew of techs who were already in the angiography suite. Annette was in the procedure room, asleep on the table. I stood next to her little body. A two-year-old has very small arteries in her legs, and I had already entered her femoral artery once before, for the previous procedure. I wanted this to be the last time I punctured that artery, because small arteries have a greater risk of scarring, which might cause her problems later with leg circulation. The challenge of being minimally invasive is magnified tremendously when the patient's body weighs less than thirty pounds. It was one of the risks I'd had to consider before deciding not to go after the DAVF in the first procedure. In the case of a child, everywhere you turn there's a risk.

I inserted the guidewire and catheter into the port I had placed in Annette's femoral artery and delicately worked it upward through the aortic arch and into her neck. The distances were so short that I felt as if I were working on a doll. The first part of the journey went smoothly, but soon it became obvious that, despite the shorter distance, reaching the DAVF itself would not be easy. I tried to guide the wire into her skull via the jugular vein on the right side, but the vein could not be accessed from below because of an obstruction. I backed the wire out and tried going up the left jugular and around the back of her head, but Annette's anatomy would not allow my catheters and wires to cross the midline of the brain. With increasing concern, I redirected my wire down another vessel and tried going through the feeding arteries in the brain, but again I could not reach the DAVF.

Four hours had gone by and I wasn't where I needed to be inside Annette's head. I was frustrated and tired of trying unsuccessfully to find a path to the DAVF. If I couldn't get my catheter near it, I couldn't treat it. I cringed every time I stepped on the pedal to beam radiation into Annette so I could see what I was doing. I didn't want this procedure to fail—another procedure would mean another puncture of her artery, more anesthetic, more wires and tubes traveling through her young vessels, more radiation. There is a limit to what surgery can do without accumulating harmful effects.

I pulled out my wire and catheter and set them on the table. I stepped back, took off my protective lead apron, and left the room for a few minutes. Except for a small port in Annette's leg, there was no evidence that I had been working for four hours on her body. Since no incision is made on the head in these procedures, taking a few minutes does not endanger the patient; in fact, to continue the procedure while frustrated or angry can often cause errors in judgment. It had become my practice, when surgery wasn't going well and I had been working for a long time without success, to step out, clear my head, drink some water, and pray. A few minutes' reprieve from the tension allows me to return to the operating table with fresh perspective and sometimes even new ideas.

I stood in the small side room drinking my water and praying, *God, what haven't I tried?* After that brief but refreshing break, I returned to Annette's side with an idea. The assistants and techs looked at me, ready, eyes alert above their masks. I decided to try my original route through the right jugular, using a stiffer wire that might push past the obstruction. I inserted the new wire, threaded it up into the right side of the neck, and after some manipulation, felt it pass farther than the other wire had. The attempt had worked. I gently pushed the wire into the back of Annette's head and into the DAVF, and I slid the micro-catheter over the wire and into the specific vein where the problem resided. It had taken me five hours, but I had reached my destination. Now came the hard part.

I took a digital subtraction angiography (DSA) of Annette's blood flow to see how quickly it was moving through the vessels. Then I stepped to the back table and mixed the glue with contrast agent and metal powder. There was a sober feeling in the room because everyone knew that this was the critical moment. It was unlikely that I could get into this position again, so I had one chance to close off the DAVF. With one swing, I had to hit a hole in one.

I stood next to Annette and got the catheter ready for the injection. Then I took the syringe and fitted the needle into the micro-catheter, then began injecting the glue. Because I was in a vein, I was injecting against the flow of blood, which made things more challenging and unpredictable. I watched as the glue began to fill the large vein on the right side of her head. The glue flowed smoothly and began to adhere to the vein. *When should I stop?* I thought. I held the syringe in my hands, pressing ever so slightly on the plunger, my eyes riveted to the screen as I watched the glue harden in the young girl's vein.

There, I thought—that was enough. I stopped, pulled suction back on the syringe, and pulled out the micro-catheter. I had made the crucial decision and there was no going back. The glue continued to harden. There was nothing to do now but see what the angiogram would show. The techs put the camera in the right place over Annette's head while I injected contrast dye and made another DSA "video." The video came up on the screen, and what I saw made my heart jump with joy. The vein had been successfully blocked, and the DAVF was almost completely eradicated. I sighed beneath my mask. Perfect. Six hours after we had begun, we had made the hole in one.

It takes time to put a child to sleep and to wake her up. Annette had been asleep for nearly eight hours and was slow to wake up. I was so fatigued, mentally and physically, that I was moving slowly myself. I caught up with her and her mother in the recovery room, where Annette was now awake and moving her arms and legs.

"Move your fingers for me," I said. She moved them beautifully.

"Now your toes," I said. She wriggled her toes. I stood up and turned to her mother, feeling elated.

"She appears to be fine," I said. Her mother just nodded, and I noticed that she was crying. It had been a long day for all of us. To my surprise, tears began to fall from my eyes as well.

"Thank you, God, for helping me in there," I prayed aloud. "Please heal this child. Amen."

It had been one of the most taxing procedures I had ever done. Exhausted, I went home and collapsed into bed early, my thoughts full of the day's events. I was sleeping deeply when my pager went off two hours later. I fumbled for it and called the number: it was the pediatrician on duty at the hospital. Annette had suddenly stopped breathing. She was placed on a breathing machine, which kept her alive, but she was nonresponsive. I leaped out of bed, pulled on some scrubs, and headed out the door.

The first CT scan showed bleeding on the right side in the cerebellum, the hindbrain. Her ventricles, the fluid-filled spaces in the brain, were enlarged and exerting pressure on the rest of her brain. Something had gone wrong, and Annette's life was now in grave danger.

A hole was drilled and a tube placed into Annette's brain to drain the fluid that was building up pressure. Annette went into emergency surgery at five in the morning to have the bone in the back of her skull removed. We hoped that it would give the cerebellum room to swell. I expected Annette to wake up once the bone was off and the pressure relieved. She did not. Later that day, Annette was still not responsive. A fresh MRI showed that there was such swelling that the hindbrain was pushing up into the main brain, a condition called upward herniation. Then I saw something I didn't want to see: the brain stem appeared to be affected. My heart sank. I knew that it would be awhile before Annette could wake up—if she would wake up. She might remain in a vegetative state for the rest of her life. There was nothing we could do but wait and see what her little body did next.

Several days went by and Annette showed no signs of neurological activity. She did not wake up and did not move. I visited with the family and discussed the gravity of the situation. They were looking to me for guidance, but I did not know what to do. I felt humbled by the events and could only shake my head in frustration, at a loss for what to suggest. We couldn't keep the breathing tube in for more than a few weeks. If her parents wanted to assure her long-term survival, we would have to do a tracheostomy—creating a more permanent breathing hole in her windpipe below the vocal cords. This would assure that she would survive, even if she was vegetative.

Our options were dwindling, and Annette was not showing any sign of getting better.

Annette's parents seemed stunned. They had known it was a serious procedure, but parents are never truly prepared to see their child in a coma, unsure if he or she will live or die. None of us had expected this. I prayed with her parents every time we met, but every day brought the same disappointment. Nothing was happening.

Though I got the impression that faith had been a small part of their lives, one day I saw Annette's father reading a Bible in Annette's room. Then word got around about Annette, and people from all over the area came to pray for her, flowing in and out of the room like lifeblood. I could see the positive effect this was having on her parents. They seemed grateful and almost mystified by the show of love and support, often offered by people they had never laid eyes on. A community they didn't know they belonged to was gathering around them in their time of need.

Annette's mother informed me that Annette's name had been put on nationwide Web-based prayer chains; thousands of people were being asked to pray for Annette and for me. That stung a bit. I was still defensive about my reputation—having my name on a nationwide prayer chain for a bleed after surgery was not good for my ego, but I quickly swallowed my pride: I had invited prayer into the process, after all. This wasn't about me; it was about Annette.

But the stress began to take its toll. Annette's mother began having early contractions and had to be confined to a wheelchair so she wouldn't go into early labor. She could stand for only a few moments at a time. Every time I saw her, from the time of the surgery on, she was in the wheelchair, often crying and saying she felt helpless at a time when her daughter needed her most.

Days went by. Despite all our prayers and all that medical science could offer her, Annette was not improving. We could not keep her on a temporary breathing tube much longer. Her parents needed to decide whether to do the tracheostomy and assure her survival on the breathing machine or to pull the tube, taking her off the machine, and see whether she would survive. They were considering both options very seriously. Given the bleak outlook for her and the debilitated state that might await her, I reasoned in my own mind that maybe God had given the family the twins at this particular time to partially offset the loss of Annette. The need to make a decision about inserting a permanent breathing tube became urgent.

Annette's mother, who had remained at her bedside day and night grieving over her firstborn, began having serious contractions. I arrived at work one morning to find that she had been admitted to the hospital. Doctors were trying to stop her premature labor, which they believed had been caused by the agony of watching Annette slowly die. It was too early to deliver the twins—their lungs were far from developed and the babies might not survive. Now all three lives were in medical danger.

I retreated into the hallway feeling gutted and hollow. We had all been on such high alert since Annette's surgery that I didn't think I could take any more bad news. I was punch-drunk after two weeks of attending Annette, and this blow put me against the ropes. Where was God in all this? Why did things continue to get worse despite all our prayers? When I got home, I collapsed facedown on the carpet of my living room floor.

"God!" I cried. "What are you doing? Haven't they suffered enough? Annette is in a coma because of my procedure, even though we prayed constantly before and after. People all over the United States are praying for Annette, and yet things are getting worse. I have done the best work I know how to do, but now this family is facing the possibility of three dead or debilitated children. Why haven't you done something? Don't you see what is happening? Where are you?"

I was worn out and angry with God, who seemed uncaring and distant. I wanted to see his power and love manifested in this situation, and it wasn't happening. I went to bed with resentment in my heart. That night I had a particularly poignant dream: The scene was a courtroom, and I was the prosecuting attorney. God was the Judge. I was standing and pointing an accusing finger at him, demanding, "Why?" Then the back doors to the courtroom opened, and Annette walked up and took the witness stand. She said only one sentence. I couldn't hear what she said, but the Judge was smiling, and I knew the case was over. I dropped my accusing finger and felt ashamed. One sentence had changed everything. Then the dream ended.

I woke up knowing that my accusing tone toward God was unjustified. In Annette's situation, as with every situation, I was missing information. It seemed so obvious to me now, so practical. I had been working without all the facts. Only God has a comprehensive view, and he is trustworthy and good. As I readied for work, I made an important decision. Though I could see no good in the situation, I could still declare that God is good. I could choose to affirm what I could not see and did not feel. I began to declare, "If I know one thing, I know that God is good." My words had the power to change my feelings: I felt more courageous and confident.

I also realized that at least some of my anger and self-pity had been in response to a bruised ego. I was angry that my long and difficult procedure had caused harm rather than good, and frustration that I could not answer Annette's family's questions about whether she would survive left me feeling inadequate. My initial response had been to blame God for the situation, which also reflected poorly on me. Now I verbally gave my reputation and the situation to God, no matter what happened. He was ultimately in charge of Annette's life—and mine.

The next time I went to the hospital, I knew I needed to change the atmosphere in Annette's room. Anger with God is not a small problem in the pediatric ICU, one of the most depressing places on the planet. As children struggle for life, attached to tubes and machines, we naturally ask, "Why?" We rarely receive an answer that satisfies. Many have lost their faith in the pediatric ICU, and I could sense among Annette's family a growing doubt that God was good. As each day passed with no sign of hope, we were all asking ourselves why God would let this happen to an innocent child.

"I was hoping that things would have changed by now," I said to them honestly as we all stood near Annette's bed, where she lay motionless and silent but for the rasping of the ventilator. It seemed altogether possible that Annette would either die or wither up, having to be turned from side to side for the rest of her life, but I kept these thoughts to myself.

"The fact that I don't know what to do is embarrassing to me, because I am supposed to know," I said. "But I know one thing. I know that God is good no matter what we see in this room. I have decided that, no matter which path we take medically with Annette, we should keep showing up and continue to declare that God is good. We will cry together and laugh together and make decisions together. And we will declare that he is good no matter what happens."

They nodded in agreement. In a crisis, it is possible, even noble, to lend others your faith. Theirs seemed to be deepening.

"Let's all gather around her and say together what we know to be true," I said. They all moved closer to the bedside and, after a short pause, repeated the short phrases I spoke. "Even though I don't understand why this is happening, . . . God, I declare that you are good. . . . You are good all the time, . . . even if I can't see it or feel it. . . . You love Annette more than we do. . . . You have Annette's best interests in mind."

When I said that God loved Annette more than we did, the words pierced my heart and I wept without shame as I heard Annette's parents proclaiming that belief through their tears. *Of course he does*, I thought. *Why didn't I think of that sooner?*

"No matter what happens," I continued to lead them, "or how long this goes on, . . . we will continue to show up. . . . We will continue to declare that you are good, . . . and we will praise you because you are worthy."

Though the little girl before us was wasting away, somehow it felt like a day of victory. The atmosphere in the room had changed. Doubt and blame were pushed back, and peace came in. We even laughed for the first time in two weeks. Instead of blaming God, we honored and declared his goodness even though we couldn't see it. We had placed Annette in God's hands. We knew that whatever happened, God was with us and with Annette. Whatever happened, it would be okay.

I walked out of that room with a new goal: to keep proclaiming that God is good even when evidence does not seem to show it. I now saw this as an opportunity that I would be crazy to miss. It took no faith to claim that God is good when life is going well. But in these circumstances it took pure, childlike faith to believe that God is good. It reminded me of the faith Annette had in me when I called her over in my office. She didn't hesitate one bit, but walked right up to me, believing my intentions toward her were only good. That was the kind of faith God was looking for in me, and in all of us. Without knowing it, Annette had taught me a lesson that was taking me through a trial that threatened her very life.

After that meeting, Annette's mother stopped having premature contractions. Her pregnancy stabilized. The family and I met again, and our peace remained. There were tears but also smiles in the room now. Sometimes we laughed together. Finally, after several more days of waiting, the family decided to take Annette's breathing tube out and not to insert a permanent one in her trachea. If God wanted her to survive, she would survive without the machine. We met together one last time and decided to remove the ventilator the following day. As I left our meeting, I saw one set of grandparents sitting on a bench in front of the hospital, holding each other and crying. It had been a long journey for all of us, but it looked as if the journey was about to end.

The next morning, with Annette's parents present, we removed Annette's breathing tube and ventilator. She now had no supplemental oxygen. We looked at her small, inert body and listened to the wicked-sounding stridor, the rasping sound that had developed due to weeks of having a plastic tube down her windpipe. I winced at the sound of it. We said nothing, but we knew what was ahead. Annette would slowly stop breathing. When she did, the family would be faced with a new challenge: to move on with their lives in the face of devastating loss. We watched in silence. Annette's oxygen monitor beeped a warning. The level of oxygen in her blood was falling. She appeared to be struggling for breath.

I turned to the nurse and told her to administer some medicines to make Annette more comfortable and help her breathe easier. She did, and her breathing became less laborious and raspy. *At least she won't have to struggle so much*, I thought. Her mother watched her somberly but with a deep peace and resolve. The grandparents looked as if someone had torn out their hearts and thrown them on the floor. I left the family there and told the nurse to call me if anything happened. She knew what I meant.

Back at my office I met with other patients, but Annette was constantly on my mind. I kept waiting to receive a call from the nurse with the bad news. The call never came. Instead, when I spoke to the nurse next, she told me that

Annette's oxygen levels had dipped only briefly, and then she had begun keeping them up without the machine.

I had a scheduled meeting out of town, and when I returned to the office, I had a message from Annette's pediatrician asking me to check on Annette. Her condition had changed. I rushed in to see the girl and her parents.

"She's slowly getting better," said Annette's father, cautiously hopeful. "She moves this arm and this leg a little, and she's been looking around the room. She seems to be tracking me with her eyes."

I looked at Annette. Her eyes were open but not exactly comprehending. She had not deteriorated as I thought she would. She had regained consciousness and was clearly fighting for life. Now she needed our help.

"She wants to live," I said. "I think we should support her."

Her father nodded. This was exactly what he wanted to hear. We did three separate shunt procedures to reroute the fluid collecting in and around her brain. People from many churches and denominations continued to stream in to pray for Annette. Friends held a fund-raiser for the family to help defray the medical costs and living expenses while Annette's father was away from his job. We all waited to see what Annette would do next.

Over the next month, Annette slowly improved. It became apparent that she might not only survive but even regain some of her brain function. A physical therapist began working with her to get her limbs moving again. Although Annette did not speak for many months, it was obvious that her mind was sharp. She answered questions by pointing to flash cards. The perceptive little girl I had first met in my office had returned.

Annette's mother soon delivered healthy twins, a boy and a girl, just down the hall from Annette's room. On Christmas Day it was decided that Annette was healthy enough to go home. Her parents took her back home with great celebration. She was introduced to her new brother and sister, and her brain function continued to improve. Three months after the surgery, she began to try to speak again. Six months after the surgery, she was learning to walk with a child-sized walker. One year later, she could walk without the walker for short periods.

When I saw Annette again for a checkup, she was still a wonderfully trusting and sensitive girl, but her personality had changed somewhat after the surgery. She'd become more assertive, bolder. She was pushing herself to walk again. Her will to survive, which had kicked in after she was removed from the ventilator, was now pushing her to do even more.

Annette's parents had changed too. The crisis and pain had shown them their need for God. Seeing the outpouring of support from the Christian community, they went from coasting through life to having a faith that could withstand a storm. When I saw them for Annette's checkups, we always spent time talking about what they were learning about God. It was as if someone had plugged them in and turned them on. Annette's crisis, for all its hardship, had changed their lives. They looked at things differently, through spiritual eyes, and they knew that God was with them.

Never again could I accuse God of being unfeeling or uncaring, because now I was certain I had no grounds to do so. I would never have all the information; only he does. My job is to work with as much skill as I can and declare that God is good in every circumstance. I might not like what he does or understand why he sometimes lets someone suffer or die—but that is his decision, not mine.

And there would be more times, like this one, when I stand amazed and watch him pull a little child back from the brink of death.

CHAPTER 10

SNATCHED
FROM HELL

CHARLOTTE WAS A MEDICAL PROFESSIONAL who worked in a hospital across town and was training to be a doctor. But she was hiding a terrible secret: her husband, Alan—a massive, muscular man—was tormented by anger and rage. He drank too much and was physically abusive toward her, even in front of their daughter and son, both under three years old.

Alan was a classic bully. Something was eating him up on the inside, and he took it out on those nearest him. He pushed Charlotte around when he felt like it. He told her she was unattractive. She suspected him of having multiple affairs. When their daughter had health problems, he arrived to her surgery drunk. On another occasion, after Charlotte

herself was discharged from the hospital following a procedure, Alan yelled at Charlotte because he had to pick her up.

Alan's abuse had been at a critical stage for a year or more.
Ashamed, Charlotte hid her bruises with clothing. She could
not believe that she, a member of the medical community,
was living life as a battered woman. Unable to bring herself
to admit her secret to anyone, she hoped that somehow Alan
would change for the better.

One night, with Alan in a drunken rage, Charlotte tried
to get him to leave the house because she feared for the children's safety. He became more violent than usual. He took
her by the hair and dragged her off the bed. Clumps of her
hair fell from his fingers, and she knew she would have to
wear a cap to work the next day to hide the damage. She
grabbed the children, locked the door, and went to bed with
an unprecedented headache.

She woke up in the wee hours of the morning feeling as if
she were dying. Her body felt "mushy," she told me later, as
if it were breaking down completely. She ran down the hall
screaming, then concluded it was just an anxiety attack. She
went back to bed with her two children.

Alan was forced to move out a week later when Charlotte
called his family and threatened to report him to the police if
they didn't intervene. The sick feeling and headaches did not
go away but worsened, leaving Charlotte partially incapacitated. She could hardly get out of bed, let alone go to work.
Her children would wake up and stare at her, wondering what
was wrong with Mommy. A friend took her to the emergency

room, but a CT scan failed to find anything. Her blood pressure was far too high, but nobody knew why. Charlotte was always careful not to mention the beatings to anyone, so the cause remained a mystery. They diagnosed her with ophthalmic migraines, gave her medicine, and sent her home.

At home, however, her symptoms grew worse. During a frightening episode of vomiting and temporary loss of vision and balance, she had to leave the kids with a neighbor while an ambulance took her to the emergency room.

An MRI showed nothing, so after two days they sent her home to recover, but the episodes of dizziness came every half hour, followed by incapacitation and vision loss. Charlotte began setting out a loaf of bread and water for the kids' meals. When she made it into work she would bump into walls, and she had lost so much weight that her coworkers were alarmed.

Finally, convinced that she was dying, she asked a medical colleague for help, and this colleague called a neurologist who ordered a scan. In the meantime, Charlotte and her children moved in with a friend.

This scan showed something: vertebral artery dissections in both arteries leading to the brain. That means the inner lining of the vessel walls had separated from the outer vessel walls in the arteries just before these two arteries enter the back of the brain. It is a dangerous condition that can cause stroke, brain damage, or death. A common cause is trauma or whiplash. Because the damage was to vessels leading to the brain, Charlotte was referred immediately to me.

I met her for the first time in my office at nine o'clock

one morning. She seemed distracted and unable to focus on one thing for very long. I started evaluating her, but she was so fatigued that she didn't seem to be paying much attention to what was happening.

"Am I going to die?" she kept repeating. "Can you fix it? I have a lot to live for. I have two little kids who need me."

Each time she said it, it was as if she didn't remember having said it before.

I looked closely at the scans. The bilateral vertebral dissections jumped out at me. Just before entering the brain, the vessels suddenly narrowed as if something had taken a bite out of both sides. I rarely see such pronounced dissections on both vertebral arteries at once.

I turned the computer screen toward her to show her the images.

"Damage like this is often caused by whiplash or a sudden, traumatic movement," I said as I looked them over. "Do you have any idea what might have happened?"

She quickly shook her head. "No," she said. "Nothing like that has happened to me."

It didn't seem entirely plausible that she would have suffered such an injury without having an idea what had caused it, but whatever the case, the important thing now was deciding on treatment. After carefully considering the options, I concluded that the risks of a procedure would outweigh possible benefits. I recommended that we let the arteries heal on their own.

"You can't do anything?" Charlotte asked, exasperated. "I can't even work or watch my children. I—I'm a wreck."

"I really am sorry," I said. "Surgery will not get you back to work any sooner and may make you worse. This is the best avenue. We will start you on blood thinners to avoid stroke until the body heals the damage. You are not to strain or pick up anything heavy. Your arteries will heal. It will just take time."

For six weeks Charlotte stayed home and suffered with her symptoms: the strange feeling that life was in slow motion, and the sudden sensation of electricity that would surge through her and rob her of the ability to see, stand, or walk straight. Eventually, I got another call from her colleague saying that Charlotte was in despair and asking whether there was anything else I could do. Although I didn't have anything else medically to offer, I was willing to give her another appointment out of compassion and a conviction that perhaps there was more to her case than what we saw in the scans.

She arrived looking distracted and distraught.

"Charlotte, we have talked about the dissections: how long they are and how the blood thinner is helping you avoid forming blood clots while your arteries heal," I said. "And we have been trying to treat your dangerously high blood pressure with limited success." I paused. "Sometimes these types of problems result from something else going on in your life, some problem that seems unrelated."

That was all it took. This woman sitting in my exam room burst out crying. There was nothing proper about it. It was messy and desperate. She looked too spent to be embarrassed, and she was too helpless to stop.

"I am so angry and bitter at my husband," she said. "I filed for divorce because he treated us horribly. He drank too much. He was mean to me and my children. He is still harassing me, calling me dozens of times a day, making threats and calling me names. I had to get a restraining order against him. He still yells at me and pushes me around when we exchange the kids."

Clearly, there was a lot going on that I didn't know about.

"Those are big problems," I said. "I think they require some serious attention and counseling. You can't leave yourself or your children in danger. In the meantime, I often pray with patients, and I would like to pray for you."

She reacted strongly.

"I grew up in church. I know about God," she said with vitriol. "Those people were hypocritical. I resent the whole concept of God. I resent my stepmother for treating me badly and claiming to be a follower of Jesus. I resent my father for letting her do it."

She paused for a moment, then dried her tears. I thought she might get up and walk out. Instead she said, "But you can pray for me."

"I meant I'd like to pray for you now," I said calmly.

"Right here? Right now?"

"Yes," I said as gently as I could, and my manner seemed to have an effect on her. She was nervous and agitated, but she seemed to feel an urgent need for something to be done. She agreed to my praying.

I scooted over on my chair.

"First, let me explain that my experience tells me that some physical problems have emotional causes," I said, explaining to her the relationship between forgiveness and health.

"Forgiveness is not pretending evil never happened, and it is not calling evil good. Forgiveness is setting yourself free by not giving others the power to hurt you again every time you think about them. Given your physical situation, it is the best way I know to help your body continue to heal."

She seemed to understand this.

"So before we pray, I think it would be a good idea for you to forgive anyone who has been hurting you."

She thought for a while.

"I need to forgive my father," she said. "He married a woman who did not love me, and he did not defend me from her. She was always against me."

"Anyone else?" I said.

This time the silence lasted longer.

"I need to forgive my husband," she finally admitted. "I feel like I married a man I didn't know."

"What do you need to forgive him for?" I asked.

"Harsh words. Suspected affairs. Drinking. Putting me down. Making me believe something is wrong with me, that I'm unattractive. Even killing my dog."

Taking it all in, I nodded.

"Then let's forgive him for those things," I said, and together we directed ourselves to God and went through the steps that were familiar to me by now, naming each offense and giving it over to him. Charlotte started crying. Her face swelled and reddened. Years of loneliness and anger seemed to be pouring out of her.

After forgiving her father and stepmother, she repeated these words in forgiveness of her husband: "I forgive Alan and I leave him in the hands of God, who is just and doesn't need my help. I drop any desire for vengeance, and I set Alan free."

I was surprised at the depth of her despair and pain, and as she continued, she embraced the process. Soon she was searching her memory as if it were an old attic, finding every bit of junk to throw away. I knew she couldn't cover it all in one visit, but already she seemed to have hope.

When we finished, she looked limp.

"How do you feel?" I asked.

"Lighter and freer emotionally," she said. "I feel better. My head still hurts a little, but I'm no longer dizzy."

"You will feel better," I said. "Give it a bit of time."

She paused.

"This feels like the beginning of something for me," she said. "I have a peace I've never had."

"That comes from God," I said. "You have just let go of a whole lot of baggage. It will try to come back, but you don't ever have to pick it up. If you feel the resentment again, just start to forgive."

She wiped her eyes. We walked out together and scheduled her for a follow-up scan.

"Thank you, Dr. Levy," she said.

• • •

Alan and Charlotte were eventually divorced. Because of Alan's continued bullying, the judge limited him to supervised visits, and after a while Alan stopped showing up at all. Charlotte didn't hear from him for five months. In the meantime, she had completed her training and was a family-practice physician. She came back for a number of follow-up appointments. I checked a scan at three months and saw that although the progress was slow, her arteries were healing. She was eager to pray the next time she saw me, and soon I referred her to two women with whom she could pray on a more regular basis. These women would pray with her, sometimes for hours. When I asked Charlotte one day how this was going, she told me they had become like the sisters she'd never had.

Her vessels healed; her symptoms decreased in severity and frequency, from fifty episodes a day to ten, then two. Finally one day in my exam room, Charlotte broke down and admitted what Alan had done to her. We were looking at her scans, and the reality of what had caused her dissections seemed to overwhelm her.

"I know how this happened," she whispered, her voice trembling. "My ex-husband . . . he would put his hands on me. One night he dragged me off the bed by my hair."

She sobbed quietly. I listened.

"He hurt me many times, bruising me, shoving me around. But this time was the worst," she said. "I think it nearly killed me."

I was not surprised to hear it. I felt a deep sadness that she had kept her secret for so long but also shared her relief that the truth was out. It is widely recognized that confession, whether in church or out, is good for the soul, and Charlotte was benefiting from it before my eyes.

"I'm so sorry for being a liar," she said. "All these people have been trying to figure out what had happened to me, and I knew all along that it was him."

She hung her head. As a member of the medical community, she was embarrassed by this revelation. I reassured her that I did not think less of her; the trauma did not change my treatment or diagnosis.

I was glad her life had taken a new direction.

• • •

Charlotte soon recovered enough to return to work full time. She was able to care for her children again. Her life became more stable with the help of a good nanny, and she hadn't heard from Alan in months. Then one day, her cell phone rang.

"Hello, this is a nurse in the intensive care unit at the hospital across town," the voice said. "Are you the ex-wife of Alan Hanson?"

After some hesitation, Charlotte replied, "Yes."

"I'm calling because Alan is extremely ill. He coded today—his heart stopped and we had to bring him back. He is awake now but is crying and would really like to see his children. Can you please bring them? I'm not sure how much time he has left."

Charlotte was torn. Should she see the man who had caused her so much misery? Should she allow him to see his children before he died? Or should she let him die alone?

What about the journey of forgiveness she had been through? What about all those offenses she had laid down? Could she really face this man who had nearly killed her? Could she do him a kindness? Should she?

She consulted with a friend at work, who recommended against it. "He doesn't deserve it after all that he has put you and the kids through," her colleague said. "He doesn't even visit them." While Charlotte waited a day wrestling with these questions, the nurse from the other hospital called back again.

"Alan is in bad shape," she said. "He keeps asking to see his children—and you."

"I'm not sure I can come," Charlotte said.

"I beg you to hear the wish of a dying man," the nurse said, "if there's any way possible."

Compassion tugged at Charlotte's heart. She composed herself and hours later walked into the intensive care unit alone. A cardiologist was walking out of Alan's room. Charlotte pulled him aside and introduced herself as Alan's ex-wife and a doctor.

The cardiologist seemed to open up in the presence of another medical professional.

"I just pulled 500 cc's of bloody fluid from the sac around his heart," he said, shaking his head. "There is massive buildup of fluid in both lungs. We've taken five liters off in the past few days. It's not looking good. He may be in his early forties, but he has the heart and lungs of an eighty-five-year-old man. He's barely hanging on."

He gave her a grim look and walked away.

Slowly, Charlotte made her way into Alan's room. The man in the bed did not look like her ex-husband. He was emaciated and weak. His eyes drifted to the door as if expecting another nurse, but when he saw it was Charlotte, his face lit up with an almost desperate recognition. He summoned his energy and waved her in.

"I'm so happy to see you," he said in a hoarse whisper.

"Alan, what's wrong?" she said. "What happened?"

"I don't know. I couldn't brush my teeth, couldn't change clothes."

He paused to take extra breaths.

"I guess it's real bad," he concluded. "Where are the kids?"

"I didn't bring them," she said. His face dimmed.

Because Charlotte was still scared of Alan and did not know in what condition she would find him, she had left the children in the waiting room. Seeing him now, she realized that Alan obviously didn't have much time left. He was only a skeleton of the large, muscular man she had known, and she was moved with compassion.

"Alan," she said. "I want you to know that I have forgiven you for all the terrible things you did to me."

He shook his head woefully as it lay on his pillow, looking as if he felt he didn't deserve to hear those words.

"I wish I could make it up to you," he said. "All the things I did to you and the kids. Everything I put you through . . ."

"Alan, you need more than my forgiveness. What you really need is God's forgiveness," she said.

He looked at her weakly.

"Okay," he said, nodding.

"Would you repeat a prayer after me?" she asked with trepidation.

"Okay," he said softly, nodding again.

"Jesus,"

"Jesus," he said flatly,

". . . I know I'm a sinner."

". . . I know I'm a sinner." This seemed to hit him harder.

"I've done terrible things to people . . . ,"

"I've done terrible things to people . . . ,"

". . . including my family."

". . . including my family." Now he was speaking from the heart. His voice broke as he continued to follow her lead: "I accept your forgiveness. Thank you for paying the price for my sins on the cross. I want to live with you in heaven forever. Amen."

He looked at her with tears in his eyes and nodded.

"Alan," she said, "I'll go get the kids."

Charlotte and the children visited his hospital room every day for the next several weeks. His condition was getting worse by the day. He was constantly short of breath. Daily he was producing a liter of bloody fluid that had to be drained from his lungs.

"Jesus, help me," he would say with labored breathing. "Lord, help me."

The doctors found a cancerous lymph node in his left groin, meaning the cancer had spread throughout his body, seeding the sac around his heart and the pleura around the lungs. One day the oncologist showed Charlotte the scans. She looked at them and cried. No part of his lung looked normal. As one doctor to another, the oncologist confided, "He's not going to make it out of the hospital."

A few days later his breathing became so compromised that he was fitted with a mask that sealed around his nose and mouth and brought pressurized oxygen into his lungs. When the children sat on his lap, they could barely see him because the breathing apparatus almost obscured his face. Nevertheless, Charlotte could see a major difference in the man who had once terrorized her. His condition had humbled him; his having received forgiveness from God and Charlotte had begun to transform him. He had even begun to compliment her whenever she was there, telling her how pretty she was. He was natural and loving with the children.

Once she was sitting quietly by his bed when he said, "By the time I finally get it and am at peace with myself and love God, he's going to take me away." He looked away with chagrin.

One day on the way to the hospital she stopped by the store to buy a CD player so she could play worship music in Alan's room. She was in the checkout line at the store when the nurse called her. "His kidneys and liver are shutting down," she said. They both knew what it meant.

At the hospital, Alan's body was cold and clammy, but his eyes were wide open. Charlotte remained calm and put on the new worship CD. He lay in bed listening to it. At one point he took a pen in hand to write a note: "How much longer?" He passed it to Charlotte.

"I don't know," she said. "But you're ready."

She left briefly to get lunch at the hospital cafeteria, and when she returned, the ward was in a frenzy. Nurses, doctors, and respiratory techs were running in and out of Alan's room, and as she walked in, he was looking at the ceiling, crying. She knew he was on his way out of this world, and she grabbed his shoulders, looked him in the eye, and said, "Alan, God loves you!" As she straightened up, a nurse watching the heart monitor announced that Alan's heart had stopped. The torso of his body rose up and then collapsed, rattling the bed. When Charlotte looked down at him, he was different than he had been seconds earlier: he was an empty shell. The green flat line and silence of the monitor told her he was gone.

Charlotte spoke at his memorial service:

For so long, Alan had a strong body but a hole in his heart. He was consumed by hatred and self-destruction. In the end his heart was made whole but his body was taken. It would have been a shame for him to die unforgiven, and I would be tormented if I had not

responded to his plea to come visit him. But every time
I think about it now, I feel peace. I did everything I
could for him.[1]

I called her the day after Alan died.

"Thank you, thank you, thank you, Dr. Levy," was all she could say. "Thank you for being faithful and taking a risk to pray and talk about spiritual things. My path toward healing started when you spoke to me about the spiritual side of health and didn't just settle for giving me blood thinners. If you hadn't helped me forgive, I would have been too bitter to see things correctly. I wouldn't have been there to tell Alan about the forgiveness that he needed from God. Your choice to take a risk changed my life, and it changed Alan's life before he died."

Charlotte continues to flourish in her relationship with God, and her children are healthy and happy. She told me recently that she prayed with a patient who had end-stage liver failure—she was able to see him receive forgiveness and peace before he died. She is a living reminder to me of what is at stake every time someone walks through my office door. Life is short, and it is full of need—sometimes desperate need. But it is just as full of opportunities to be used by God in astonishing and eternal ways.

CHAPTER 11

WHEN
COMPLICATIONS ARISE

It is one thing to pray for good outcomes or to lead patients through forgiveness for the sake of their health. It is an entirely different thing, and much more difficult, to accept God's forgiveness when procedures I perform result in injury.

Ken, a thirty-year-old man, came to me with a benign tumor behind his forehead. His operating surgeon wanted me to cut off the blood supply to it so that it would bleed less during the tumor-removal procedure—and he wanted it done the following day. I planned to do this the way I usually do, by gluing shut the vessels that feed the tumor. It promised to be a straightforward procedure, but initially when I met with Ken and his wife, he told me he did not want it done. That surprised me, and I assumed it was typical patient apprehension. I didn't put any pressure on him but discussed the possible benefits versus risks. With his wife's encouragement, by the end of the appointment he had come around to the idea and agreed to do it. I added his case to the schedule and was confident that it would go well.

On the day of the procedure I prayed with Ken in pre-op, and before the procedure I prayed with the technologists who would be helping me. Ken was placed under general anesthesia, and I joined him in the procedure room where he was unconscious and draped in blue. My techs were ready. So was I.

I had seen the vascular tumor on the MRI, but as with many other procedures, I wouldn't know exactly what the vessels feeding the tumor looked like until the procedure began. To see the vessels clearly, I needed an angiogram. I guided the small plastic tube from his femoral artery to the carotid artery in his neck, injected contrast dye, and did an angiogram. The movie, showing dye flowing through the tumor, came up on the screen. The vessels taking blood into the tumor behind his eye were obvious. The tumor was also invading the base of his skull. There was something else, though: the same vessels that supplied blood to the tumor were also supplying blood to the skin of his face. That was troublesome. It immediately elevated the risk from moderate to high. I stopped the procedure.

I often do pre-operative embolization procedures for other surgeons, preparing the tumor for easier removal. Since the other surgeons are the primary ones in these cases, whenever there is a serious question, I want them involved in the decision. It usually comes down to who will take the risk: them or me.

"Get Dr. Miller on the phone," I said to one of the techs as I headed toward the reading room. Within moments, Ken's primary surgeon was on the line.

"I just looked at the angiogram, and the same vessels that supply the tumor also supply the skin of the face," I said. "I'm seeing real danger to his facial skin if we go through with this. I suggest we not do the embolization."

I heard silence on the other end, and I knew Dr. Miller was going to take the opposite view. He wanted me to plug up the vessels so he would have a cleaner surgery, and I didn't blame him. Bloody tumor removals are more risky to perform because you often can't see what you're cutting out. There are a lot of nerves at the base of the skull, where the tumor was invading.

"I think you can do it," he said. "That tumor is large. It is a tricky area to operate in and I don't want it to bleed. I also don't want to transfuse him. C'mon, Dave, you can do it. You're a star."

"Well, I appreciate the confidence," I said. "But I'm not sure the benefits are worth it."

"I disagree," he said. "I have complete confidence in you, and I think it's the right course of action. I don't want this thing bleeding all over when I go in to remove it. If you can see any way to do it, I encourage you to give it a try."

We hung up, and I considered my position. Why was this new wrinkle troubling me but not my colleague? Was I just having an off day? being too skittish? One of the techs came over to sound out what I was thinking.

"I'm not comfortable with it," I explained. "The risk is going to be higher than I expected, and I have a hard time justifying it compared with the possible benefits."

"Nah, you could do this, easy," he said. "You've had tougher cases. You can get up there and close those vessels. This could be over in thirty minutes. Why not give it a try?"

The techs had tremendous faith in my abilities. They had seen me do hundreds of procedures, and we had failed relatively few times together. The others watched me from their posts around the room. I was the only one hesitating. Perhaps I was wrong. Everybody else believed in my skills, why didn't I? A familiar feeling came over me—the desire to be the hero in this situation, to help this man in a way few people could. After all, this was what I'd been trained for.

I tried to shake off my doubt.

"All right," I said. "Let's do it."

Everyone snapped back to action. The show was on.

I inserted the micro-catheter through the guide catheter positioned in Ken's neck. I proceeded up the external carotid artery and soon encountered my first problem—a tortuous twist in the vessel. Though I was using the smallest catheters and wires available, the path to get into position proved to be an obstacle course. There were corkscrew turns in the vessel, and when the catheter made its way slowly through the looping area, the vessel spasmed, seizing the catheter and cutting off blood supply.

"Spasm," I said. "Get the vasodilator."

The techs went to their tasks.

Spasm of the arteries is common, especially in smaller vessels. When something such as an instrument irritates a vessel wall, a muscular reaction causes it to clamp down on the instrument. It happens in vessels of all sizes, but in the smaller vessels it can actually shut down a procedure for a time. Like a tanker caught in a frozen ocean, you have to wait for the passageway to relax in order to free up your instruments to move forward.

Thankfully, this vessel was not the only one supplying blood to that part of the body, so the lack of blood flow would not harm Ken. I injected a vasodilator to help relieve the spasm, and then we stood by in silent frustration. It was like being asked in the middle of battle to stand around and wait.

Ten minutes later the vessel had relaxed enough to move the catheter again. I proceeded gingerly through the corkscrew, past the junction where vessels branched off to supply the face, and down the vessel that went through the skull to feed the tumor. The nearby presence of the vessels feeding the face still made me uneasy. Whenever you inject glue, there is a chance that it can go the wrong way and cause serious problems. The beauty and the danger of glue is that it permanently blocks any vessels into which it is injected. Proper placement means the difference between closing diseased vessels and injuring healthy ones.

Ken's vessels were very small, so small that even with machine magnification it was difficult to see everything I was doing. I had earlier considered using not glue but little plastic particles, which go in and jam up the circulation, blocking the vessel by acting more like a dam. I chose glue in the end because the particles could also jam the small catheter I was using and not reach the target. Glue is also easier to see under X-ray and is therefore more accurate. In a complicated situation such as this, with a "good" facial vessel sitting so close to the "bad" tumor vessels, I had to be as accurate as possible.

The level of complication still bothered me as I readied the injection. I knew it would be hard to control the glue in a space that small. The danger was that I would push too much glue in at once, causing it to flow back up the vessel and into the branch supplying the face. To make it more difficult, the X-ray machine was having trouble seeing down to that level. I could still see what I was doing but was now working at the limits of the machine's visualization capabilities.

My catheter sat in the vessel supplying the tumor, past the branches supplying the face. I had mixed the glue and put it into the syringe. I did a practice run with contrast dye to watch the flow into the tumor. It went briskly. There was nothing left to do but inject the glue.

With a screw-type motion I attached the glue syringe to the back end of the micro-catheter, which was sitting on the blue drape overlaying Ken's knee. I said, "Blank road map," and the tech next to me pressed a button to change the function of the machine. I stepped on the pedal, and the screen went blank—a light gray tone. This screen would register only the movement of the glue as it flowed into the tumor instead of showing all the other background structures.

I began to inject the glue and focused my gaze at the tip of my micro-catheter on the screen . . . and waited. Several seconds passed as the glue traveled the length of the micro-catheter. I expected it to appear as a black substance on the screen. As the breathing machine gave Ken a breath, his head moved slightly, making several areas on the screen turn black. Then I saw something appear on the screen, a darker shade of gray that seemed to be going into the tumor. It was the glue. I injected a little more, focusing on getting it deep into the tumor. Pleased that the glue was flowing as planned, I pushed the plunger more. One second, perhaps two; then in a fraction of a second I saw the glue flash back along the catheter, past the branch point for the vessels leading to the skin. I stopped injecting and quickly pulled the catheter out of the vessel before the glue hardened it permanently in place.

I exhaled forcefully. I had forgotten to breathe again.

The glue had come back a bit, but I was happy with the penetration into the tumor. The blood loss at Dr. Miller's surgery would be minimal.

Through the guide catheter still in Ken's neck, we did a final angiogram. The tumor looked like a ghost; the glue had cut off its blood supply. Feeling relieved at the success of the procedure, I left the techs to pull out the catheter and hold pressure on the puncture site until it stopped bleeding. This usually took fifteen minutes and was easier to do with the patient still asleep. A bandage over the entry point in his artery would be the only reminder of the procedure, I hoped.

Half an hour later I was reviewing the scans that showed that the vessels to the tumor had been destroyed. I was pleased with myself for having gone through with it.

"Good job, crew," I said, and the techs voiced congratulations back to me.

I stepped into a small anteroom to write orders for the nurses to carry out for Ken in the recovery room and ICU. Then the anesthesiologist called me back into the procedure room. He was removing Ken's breathing tube but had stopped to observe something.

"Look at this facial skin. It doesn't look right," he said, pointing to Ken's cheek. There, an area the size of a silver dollar had become unnaturally white. The skin was blanching. I'd seen this happen before, but never on so big an area.

"Oh God, please, no," I thought.

A feeling of horror and sickness swept over me as I quickly imagined what must have happened: glue had closed the vessels feeding the skin of his face.

"If there was an embolization of the skin, it's going to be painful," I told the anesthesiologist. "Be ready with some morphine."

A nurse rushed away to get the morphine, and I immediately went out of the room to call the plastic surgeon. Closing the blood supply to the skin is similar to frostbite. With frostbite, the blood vessels in the tips of your fingers or nose freeze, so the skin no longer receives oxygen, and it stings. If the nerves in the skin go without oxygen for more than a few minutes, they begin screaming that something is wrong—that the tissue is not getting oxygen. For the patient, this registers as one continuing cascade of pain.

In the same way, embolizing Ken's facial vessels cut off blood and oxygen to the skin. Now the nerves were clanging like a four-alarm fire bell to alert the brain that the skin was dying.

The plastic surgeon said she was on her way, and she told me to apply a topical cream to the wound, which would dilate the vessels and perhaps increase the blood supply. I went back to Ken, who was still unconscious, and applied the cream to the whitening area. The anesthesiologist gave him some morphine. Then he was wheeled up to the recovery room.

Fifteen minutes later, Ken awoke in terrible pain and began screaming and writhing in his bed. I arrived with the plastic surgeon, and we tried to observe the damaged area amid Ken's semiconscious moaning and thrashing. It was tough to get a long look at it, but the plastic surgeon agreed that the skin looked damaged.

"We won't know how bad it is for a few days," she said. "There's nothing we can do except wait and see how large it gets."

"The white part seems to be growing," I said dolefully.

"It doesn't matter what turns white," she said. "It matters what turns black."

As we left the room, I realized there might be another complication. Because the vessels were so close to Ken's eye, if there were connections, the glue may have traveled into these vessels as well. Not only was the skin on his face dying, but if the glue had traveled far enough, he might be facing blindness in that eye.

It is difficult to explain the condition I was in at that point, knowing that my procedure had caused pain and damage of this magnitude. I prayed something like, "God, . . . help," but I felt totally alone. The unexpected had happened, and there were steep consequences. I had criticized other doctors for exactly this kind of result before, citing their poor training and lack of judgment. How could I have done the same thing? How could I have gone forward, ignoring my gut instinct? How could I have listened to others instead of to myself? Had I lost my skills, my edge, my judgment? As a result of my actions, Ken might never look the same and might have only one working eye.

I can't believe I did this! I thought. I felt lightheaded, and a wave of nausea swept over me as I tried to grasp what I had done. I had no time to address my own emotions, however. Ken's family were now facing a medical crisis, and they would look to me for leadership. I tried to pull myself together before I headed to the waiting room to talk with Ken's wife and parents. They were there, tense and expectant. I took a deep breath.

"I was able to get the tumor's blood supply, but one of the risks we talked about, harming some of the skin on his face, did happen," I said. I saw them wince.

"There is going to be some damage," I continued. "I'm

just not sure how much. There also might be some loss of vision. Ken is in pain right now, but I'd like you to come with me to see him."

As I led them to the recovery room, I heaped judgment on myself. How could I have let this happen? The guilt was overwhelming.

We arrived at Ken's bay in the recovery room. He was moaning in pain. The nurses had sedated him enough to stop his thrashing, but the normal doses of morphine were barely effective. We could not give him higher doses because it might stop his breathing.

His wife rushed to his side and began stroking his head. Ken's eye was swollen shut and the white cream highlighted the wounded part of his face. With their help I calmed him down and separated his eyelids with my fingers to conduct a brief vision test.

"Ken, can you see my hand?" I asked.

He moaned. "My head hurts. It hurts so bad."

"Can you see how many fingers I'm holding up?" I asked.

He shook his head. "I can't."

The morphine took effect and he lapsed back into a stupor. I looked at his wife and parents.

"I can't tell. We'll have to wait and test him later," I said. "I would like to pray for him."

They nodded their approval, and I put my hand on his head. This prayer was for Ken but also for me. I needed to talk to God about this awful situation I had caused.

"God, we know that you are here even if we can't feel you

right now," I prayed. "We know that you love Ken, and we pray for Ken's skin and eye to heal."

I paused. I was asking God to undo the damage I had just caused, to fix supernaturally something I had done. He wasn't under any obligation to help me, and I wasn't sure it was appropriate to ask. Still, I continued out of sheer faith.

"We pray for peace—for all of us," I concluded. "In Jesus' name, Amen."

The emotional agony I was feeling made it difficult to say the words. Instinctively I knew that appealing to God was the right thing to do. It wasn't about me; it was about helping Ken.

After we prayed, I left them together and went back to my office. It was late afternoon, but I couldn't bring myself to go home. Leaving the hospital felt like a betrayal of Ken and his family. I stayed late doing paperwork and keeping busy doing nothing of significance as a sort of penance. I checked on Ken several times and applied more topical cream to his face. It was a further act of penance, since this was something the nurses normally do, and I performed it knowing all the while that it probably was having no effect; the vascular damage had been caused from the inside. In spreading the cream on his face, I was just trying to make myself feel better.

I finally went home that night and entered a weeklong nightmare of regret and self-condemnation. I was unable to eat for days, unable to think of anything else for more than a few minutes. Ken was constantly on my mind. I could not believe that I had injured his face so badly that he would need plastic surgery to reconstruct it and that I had perhaps robbed him of sight in one eye. There was nothing I could do to take it back or fix it. I replayed the tape of the procedure in my mind as if reliving some personal trauma. I had known the risk, but never before had a cosmetic outcome of this scope resulted from a procedure I had done. Fears chased through my mind: fears that I was not a good doctor, that I would lose my job, that Ken and his family would be angry with me and sue me. When I had felt hesitation during the case, I reasoned now that God had been telling me to stop. If he had been, I hadn't listened, and I had hurt a man who trusted me. I also remembered that Ken initially had not wanted the procedure.

Along with the fear, irrational anger washed over me—anger at myself, as well as at the other doctor and the technologist for encouraging me to proceed when they knew I was uncomfortable doing so. I realized anew and with awe how thin is the margin between doing great good and doing great harm in my profession. The glue was just one example of that; all the tools of brain surgery must be used within a very narrow range, and with sometimes superhuman precision. Otherwise, those tools become instruments of destruction.

I woke up the day after the surgery and each subsequent day hoping that it had all been a dream. One night I actually dreamed that it had not happened at all, only to wake up to the reality that when I arrived at the hospital, I would look under Ken's bandage—and relive the nightmare.

I checked on him three times a day. The affected area of

his face turned white, then gray. They had moved him to ICU, where a nurse kept up with his demand for narcotics. Only a strong sedative kept his pain under control. The pain would subside when the injured tissue actually died.

With each visit I would talk with his wife and family, give them—and myself—a pep talk, or console them as needed. Once his pain was under control, Ken seemed to appreciate my coming by to pray with him. I was there to be his cheerleader. His wife and parents also looked to me for assurance and guidance. They were trying to support Ken, and this was just the first step. His tumor still had to come out, and the other doctor was already scheduling the next surgery. Ken's family stayed remarkably steady throughout. We prayed together whenever they were in the room; they told me they greatly appreciated this.

It took a week before we knew that Ken's eye had not been damaged. The blurriness had been temporary and perhaps due to swelling around the eye. Unfortunately, his facial skin did not improve. On day three a small central area of the wound began turning black. This black spot spread outward until it encompassed the whole area that had initially been white. Black is a color that does not exist in the human body; it is the color of death.

Not only would plastic surgery be necessary, but Ken's face would never look like it had before.

As Ken went through his own painful recovery, I began to untangle the knot of regret and try to make sense of what I had done. The question I asked God was not, "Why do you allow suffering?" but "Why did you let it come by my hand?"

As I spun myself into ever-deeper tunnels of remorse, I knew the only path out was to follow the steps I had taught others: confess my sins to God, receive his forgiveness, and then apply his grace to what I had done. This advice seemed inadequate to the offense now that the offense was my own. Forgiveness was easy when I was prescribing it for someone else. Now I had to take my own medicine and believe that receiving God's forgiveness would help me heal.

I called a friend, a surgeon and a follower of Jesus, the kind of friend who would be especially helpful at a time like this. Most friends, especially doctors, were telling me things to make me feel better: "It is part of the risk of surgery. The patient knew the risks." "Everyone has complications." "You just need a vacation." "You have done so many great cases; focus on those." All were common expressions from sympathetic colleagues. Though having people speak to me in this way was comforting, I was in a prison of guilt and couldn't get free. I told my friend what had happened and that I was so upset I was unable to eat.

"Guilt is powerful. You're beating yourself up mentally, and your body is just following along and punishing itself," he said.

"I can't believe I did that injection. I ignored my own reservations," I said.

"You feel guilty—and maybe you are; maybe you're not," he said. "Confession is what I recommend. There is nothing that God won't forgive. Even if you confess to something you didn't do, God knows, and it can't hurt anything but your pride. Whatever you've done, it doesn't change the way God sees you, and it doesn't change the way I see you."

With my friend listening, I confessed to God what I had done, and I received God's forgiveness. Because God had forgiven me for what I had done, to continue to punish myself would mean that my standard was higher than God's. Only pride had prevented me from believing that I was forgiven. Still, my mind kept rehearsing that fateful decision to proceed, and it took awhile to feel forgiven. It became a daily battle. Each day when I walked into Ken's room, I had to remind myself that God loved me regardless of my performance.

Although I conveyed to Ken and his family how sorry I was that this complication had occurred, in this case I did not think it would be helpful to them to ask their forgiveness for the bad outcome. It was, after all, a risk of the procedure. I prayed with Ken for healing and for the upcoming tumor surgery. The only good result of my procedure was that the tumor would bleed little when they took it out.

It is mandatory to present a report to the chief of neurosurgery about any complication that takes place during surgery, and I did so. Since the complication was cosmetic and had no neurological impact on the patient, he didn't think it worthy of discussion. To me, though, the outcome was far from acceptable.

Ken went home on day seven, taking mild pain medicine.

The tumor was successfully removed two weeks later, and plastic surgery was performed at the same time to repair the damage to his face. A permanent scar remains.

A scar also remains on my heart.

• • •

The very next patient I treated was Lisa, a fifty-year-old hairstylist who required an embolization on a cigar-shaped tumor that ran along the base of her skull just behind her right ear. It was an uncommon location for a tumor and was threatening the brain stem and ear region and the nerves in that area. It was also an uncommon type of tumor and one that was bound to be bloody if the skull base surgeon tried to remove it without my first blocking the vessels.

All tumors are parasites, poaching the body's normal circulation in order to feed themselves. A tumor actually secretes a substance that causes vessels to grow into the tumor to feed it blood. The vessels supplying the tumor become enlarged, and the blood that should be going elsewhere serves to grow the tumor.

Among tumors there is great variety in the amount of vascularization, or the extent to which a tumor has taken over the blood vessels. Some tumors are avascular (having few vessels) and grow slowly. Others, like the one this patient had, are highly vascular, with a high density of vessels in and around the tumor.

On the initial scans I could see a number of normal vessels

that had been drawn in to serve the tumor. The mass was so vascularized that it was almost nothing but blood vessels, many of which were very small. It was obvious why skull base team members Dr. Samuels and Dr. Bronson wanted me to cut off the circulation of the tumor before they removed it. Bleeding in that area of the head can be profuse and can complicate surgery and require transfusions. The unusual location of the tumor also meant it sat near cranial nerves going to the ear, tongue, throat, and face. The tumor had grown around some of these nerves, making it easy to injure one of them during a bloody surgery.

Skull base surgeons know the course of the cranial nerves, carotid arteries, and other important structures that are hidden in the bones of the face, ear, and occipital region, where the skull attaches to the cervical spine. Using a drill, they shave the bone surrounding the nerves to a paper-thin layer in order to carefully separate nerve from tumor. The cases are long and tedious, more so even than typical neurosurgical cases. Removing tumors from between the cranial nerves at the base of the skull requires a level of skill, patience, and dedication that few surgeons possess.

Lisa was from out of town and had made a fairly long trip to San Diego for a double procedure: the embolization one day, followed by surgery two days later by my colleagues. I put on my hat and mask and headed into the procedure room. She was anesthetized and on the table, and I did a quick angiogram by entering at the femoral artery and navigating to the carotid artery in her neck. I went into the control room, took off my gloves, and sat down to take a look at the movielike angiogram. What I saw made me uncomfortable. As I had suspected, the vessels feeding the tumor were dangerously close to the facial nerve, which runs near the ear canal. I called Dr. Samuels, and he came down in minutes.

"This tumor is really close to the facial nerve," I said, watching the angiogram as I spoke. "I don't want to give her a facial nerve palsy."

He was silent for a few moments.

"I don't want this thing to bleed," he said. "The last time you used particles, it bled a lot. Use that new glue, the thick stuff. That works great."

He looked at his watch. There was some urgency in his schedule, and he wanted my procedure to be done that day. I looked at the angiogram again, then looked over at Lisa, unconscious and ready for the embolization. I felt immense compassion and wanted the best for her. The techs stood nearby, ready and eager to work. The train was moving down the track. Once again, I was the only one threatening to stop the momentum.

"Let me make a quick phone call," I said, and excused myself. Dr. Samuels made a sound of exasperation behind me. The techs held their places quietly.

At Dr. Samuels's request I was using a different substance, an agent that is not actually a glue but acts like one and is injected as a liquid. This black mixture has the consistency of thick molasses and is much thicker than the glue I normally use, which is thin and flows with the blood into the tumor.

You literally push this substance forward until it fills the whole tumor, vessel by vessel. It contains metal powder, which settles in the vessel and plugs it up. I had used it before, but not in this particular location. I wanted to be completely sure that there was not some history of complications with the facial nerve when using it in this part of the body. I had read a journal article that reported success in treating a large series of tumors using the glue to cut off the blood supply; it reported no major nerve injuries with it, but I could not tell whether the surgeon had been treating a similar tumor in a similar location.

I ducked into the reading room and dialed a few colleagues to run the situation by them and get their professional opinions. No one was available. The only person available was a sales representative who couldn't get company consultants on the line. Nobody knew if it was safe to use around the facial nerve.

I was going to have to make this decision on my own.

Because blood vessels supplying the facial nerve are very small and the substance is relatively thick, I reasoned that the danger of damage to the nerve was small. There was a risk, but I wasn't sure if the risk was high enough to stop the case. Maybe I was being overly cautious because of what had happened with Ken. Maybe this procedure would even offer me redemption. I had done riskier procedures before with success.

In fact, I had made a career of tackling risky problems, and the vast majority of the time it paid off. If I didn't take on this problem, Dr. Samuels would have a much more difficult surgery. The risk was his or mine to deal with.

I walked back into the procedure room.

"Okay," I said. "Let's go."

Dr. Samuels smiled and went back to his office.

I stood next to Lisa and carefully guided a catheter up her femoral artery and into her ear region. I identified three separate vessels that were feeding the tumor, selected them for embolization, and began filling them with the tarlike glue. For five hours I pushed it through the vessels and watched my progress on the twenty-four-inch screen. The images were regularly refreshed and showed the glue oozing into different parts of the tumor. The screen did not depict any body structures, including the tumor or the brain; I had to imagine where important structures were by watching the glue so I could stop the injection before it blocked important vessels.

There was one main danger I was trying to avoid. I didn't want the glue oozing down a wrong vessel, where it could get into general circulation and cause a stroke. I was constantly trying to stay within what I considered to be the boundaries of the tumor. This required me to visualize in my own mind the shape of the tumor and where it ended. If I saw the glue approaching what looked like a "normal" vessel, I stopped injecting.

Some procedures are long but fulfilling. This one was just long. In the back of my mind I was constantly thinking about the higher-than-normal risk. I knew I could cut off the tumor from its blood supply, but I was not at all sure that I could do it without causing harm, and that put me on edge.

When I finished, I was pleased with what I had done. The glue hadn't gone into the brain and didn't appear to have gone anywhere I hadn't expected it to. The scans showed that I had blocked the tumor's feeding vessels. My team of techs felt confident and happy. So did I.

It took awhile for Lisa to wake up, which was normal for a procedure that long, and when she did, I went into the procedure room to visit her. She was still groggy as I performed the usual post-operative checks.

But when I asked her to smile, only the left side of her mouth went up.

"Try again," I said. Again, she half smiled.

"Close your eyes," I said.

Her right eye would not close.

My heart sank. The facial nerve was not working. *Not another complication in the same week!* I thought. *This can't be happening.*

Since she was groggy, she did not realize that there was a problem, so I just smiled back and told her I would see her in the recovery room when she was more awake to discuss the procedure.

As I entered the case in the computer, a task required by hospital protocol for every surgery, I went over in my mind what might have caused part of her mouth not to move and an eye not to close. There had been no topical anesthesia to immobilize the face. It might have been merely the solvent in the glue that had stunned the facial nerve, meaning that it should recover. But clearly, the most obvious reason was that my injection into the vessels of the tumor had somehow traveled into the tiny nerve-feeding vessels and cut off the blood supply to the facial nerve.

Before accepting this possibility, I went to the recovery room to visit Lisa again. She was much more awake now. She perked up when I walked into her bay.

"You seem to be doing well," I said.

"I feel pretty good," she said.

"Can you smile for me?" I asked casually. She did. The same side of her mouth did not move. I noticed, too, that when she blinked, her right eye did not close completely. The injury was still there, which meant that it was more likely to be permanent.

Calmly, I said, "Lisa, there is some weakness in your face, but I don't know if it is temporary or permanent. For now, just rest. We'll talk about it later."

"Okay, Doctor," she said, seeming unconcerned. She was already looking ahead to her next surgery to remove the tumor, and for now my news was lost amid her other concerns.

I knew it was no minor concern. Back in my office, I sat alone and faced the devastating facts: a procedure of mine had injured another patient the same week in which Ken had been injured. Technically Lisa's procedure had been a success, but it also had harmed her face. Having half of your face paralyzed is significant. I had proceeded when I had reservations—again.

I leaned forward and put my head in my hands. Two complications in one week were more than I was used to having, and it stung my ego. I struggled again with self-condemnation. Would I do more harm?

Lisa went to surgery two days later and her tumor was successfully removed. The skull base team was very pleased with the lack of bleeding during the long and difficult surgery. Dr. Samuels told me that he had found the new glue in the small vessels around the facial nerve, confirming that my procedure had caused the facial nerve injury. Lisa went on to recover partial function of her face, including the ability to close her eye. Unfortunately, the right corner of her mouth didn't go up; the procedure had permanently altered her smile. Dr. Samuels also noted that if I had not done such aggressive work, the bleeding would have prevented him from seeing the facial nerve and he might easily have cut it during the surgery. Here was the blessing of teamwork; celebrating our successes and supporting one another when complications arise.

Bad outcomes are part of the medical profession. My medical diagnosis and technique will never be perfect every time. I am human, and I make errors. Still, it was painful to make rounds that included a woman who could not move half of her face and who was only two doors down from a man whose facial skin was turning black. Like anyone else, I would rather see my successes than my failures. Some physicians don't allow injured patients access to their offices. I have always thought that care of the patient and family after a bad outcome says more about a doctor than the plaques on his or her wall.

Nevertheless, I had caused two injuries in the same week. I was obviously not doing something right.

• • •

A few weeks later I was scheduled to do a procedure on Neera, an eight-year-old girl whose left hand and forearm were mildly swollen because of the AVM (Arteriovenous Malformation) located there. She was having only mild symptoms, but I was concerned that the problem might get worse. Because treating AVMs is my specialty, I occasionally treat them in odd places—such as feet, knees, hands, and tongues—and this time I would be operating on the hand. Hand AVMs are rare and difficult, and Dr. Fitzgerald, a specialist in peripheral vascular problems, came to lend his wisdom to the case. He had assisted me several times and I had learned to trust his skill and judgment: he was good.

I went into the procedure more wary than I had been in a long time. I almost distrusted my own judgment, which is a dangerous thing for someone in my position. With Dr. Fitzgerald present, I prayed with the techs and staff before starting the procedure. When I asked God for wisdom and judgment, I meant it as I had never meant it before.

I got the catheter into a good position in Neera's hand and was ready to inject the glue into her vessels and close part of the malformation.

"We're in position. What do you think?" I asked Dr. Fitzgerald, who could see from his position behind me the anatomy of her hand on the large TV monitor.

"Looks good. Glue it," he said.

I stood up and went to the back table to mix the glue,

but while performing that task, I had a feeling that moving forward was not a good idea. I stopped mixing. I wanted more time to decide.

I wrestled within myself. Was I simply losing confidence in my abilities? Was this all a mind game? Or was my better judgment speaking to me? Might it even be God giving me wisdom?

I went back to the table to stare across Neera at the angiogram again.

"You know, I want to think this through for a minute," I said to Dr. Fitzgerald. He looked at me without blinking. The techs also looked on. I felt the familiar pressure from everyone in the room. We had a child under anesthesia; this was no time to sit back and contemplate our approach. I was trained to make snap decisions, and it was time to make one.

But something didn't feel right, and this time I decided I wasn't going to ignore it.

I looked at the scans and saw nothing definitive. I looked at where the catheter was. I thought about the mixture it would require, the amount of blood flow going through those vessels, and where the glue might end up. I could not pinpoint one particular thing that disconcerted me, but I knew deep inside that it would be wrong to go ahead with treatment.

"I can't do it. I don't think it is a good idea," I finally said.

Dr. Fitzgerald just stood there blank-faced. The techs paused a moment to see if I was serious. I left the catheter in place, just in case I changed my mind again. Stopping

without treating a patient is one of the most frustrating decisions a surgeon can make, for both the doctor and the crew.
I got up, pulled off my gloves, and walked into the console
room. Dr. Fitzgerald followed me wordlessly.

Over the next few minutes, Dr. Fitzgerald and I further
explored the angiograms. There we discovered something we
had not seen before: because of a previous treatment, Neera's
thumb had an unusually poor blood supply. She had only
one artery supplying it, instead of the usual two. My injection could have easily blocked the only feeding artery, causing her to lose the thumb.

We looked at the angiogram in silence for a while. Joy
flooded over me. By not treating her, I had likely saved her
thumb.

"Good call," Dr. Fitzgerald finally said.

Half an hour later Neera woke up and moved her hand
normally, as she had before the procedure. I went home feeling humbled and relieved, mostly for Neera's sake but also
for my own. I had had every excuse to move forward with
treatment, including the encouragement of Dr. Fitzgerald,
who was more experienced in hand problems than I. But
this time I had listened to my gut—or was it God? Given
the outcome, I think it was God. The swelling in Neera's
hand and forearm persisted for the next few years but did
not increase. It would be three years before Neera would
need further treatment of her hand, and her thumb would
not be at risk during that time.

It is never easy making decisions in matters concerning

life and limb. Patients rarely know how a doctor suffers when injury happens because of a medical or surgical intervention. Even so, I know that God is always with me, as he is with the patients I serve—even when a procedure goes wrong.

None of us are beyond his grace.

CHAPTER 12

MEMORABLE CASES

BLESSING PATIENTS and addressing their emotional and spiritual health were making a world of difference for them and for me. A few cases stood out from the rest.

A woman in her late twenties named Claudia came in to see me. This pale young woman seemed unhappy, and her tone was rather whiny. Her MRI scans showed a small feature in her brain that had been labeled an aneurysm but had turned out to be nonthreatening. The reason she had gotten the scan in the first place was because of long-standing and severe headaches, the cause of which nobody could diagnose. When the small bump on her vessel showed up on an MRI, her neurologist sent her to me. Claudia was hoping that fixing the bump would help her headaches. The variation in her vessels was normal, though; there was nothing wrong with them.

Having a diagnosis of "brain aneurysm" and a visit to a neurosurgeon sometimes serves to validate a patient's mysterious headaches and to justify ongoing health concerns with family and friends. Even the words *brain surgery* can give an odd sense of comfort to someone who feels overlooked and undervalued, but I hoped to offer her something more substantial.

I began interviewing Claudia as she sat in my exam room.

"How long have you had these headaches?" I asked.

"A long time. As long as I can remember," she said.

"How would you rate the pain, on a scale of one to ten?"

"Sometimes an eight. Sometimes a five."

"What is it now?"

"Eight."

"Does it ever go away?"

"Not entirely."

In our brief exchange she had already struck me as being one of the occasional patients who bounces around the medical system but never finds a real solution for her problems. It seemed to me that medicine had nothing to offer her, and yet I also felt great compassion for her. She seemed frustrated with her life, lost somehow. I wanted to try to help her identify the real source of her trouble, whatever it might be.

We looked at the MRI together, and I told her that there was nothing of significance to the bump on her artery. It was not a true aneurysm, and there was nothing more to be done for it.

"However, you are much more complex than your MRI scan shows. There is more to you than what we can see on these studies. How are your relationships?" I asked. "Anything giving you stress?"

She exhaled slowly. "What do you mean? Like, at work or home?" she asked.

"Anywhere," I said. "Are there any people in your life making you angry?"

"Yes, I guess so," she said. "I have a terrible relationship with my mother. She drives me crazy. We haven't spoken in six months. Then my father just moved out of the country with another woman. He is worse than my mother. I don't speak to him, either."

She looked at me curiously, wondering what this had to do with her brain problem.

"I ask because negative emotions can have physical consequences, not just emotional ones," I said. "Were you raised with a faith or religion?"

"I was raised Catholic," she said, then with an air of defiance added, "but I don't believe there is a God."

I took a deep breath. This might be like trying to take a thorn out of a lion's paw. I needed to proceed very carefully. I raised my eyebrows and nodded to indicate that I had noted her anti-God sentiments and that I made no judgment of her.

"When did you decide there wasn't a God?"

"When I was nine."

"Did something happen when you were nine?"

She paused momentarily. "I was molested." She shrugged her shoulders and said it casually, as if trying to convey that it no longer affected her. But everything about her posture and expression let me know that it still hurt and that she had been living with this bitterness. Like many other people who are hurt, she had made certain choices to protect herself from further injury. *If God won't protect me, I will not believe in him*, many people think. *If God won't answer my prayers, I will do what I want with whomever I want.* These decisions feel justified at the time, but lead people to a prison of loneliness, fear, shame—and often physical illness. There is no lasting peace apart from our Creator. Sure, we can have some great highs, but none of us were designed to live apart from God.

In that moment I had hope for Claudia, and it appeared to me that this might be a divine appointment. I did not know how much she was willing to confront. Telling her the truth in a way that she could hear it was a delicate job. I had no sense that Claudia wanted to return to her faith, and I was not going to push her. One thing was clear, though: bitterness was stealing the joy from her life, and she needed help removing it.

"I'm very sorry about what happened when you were nine," I said. "A lot of people would be angry with God and would be asking why he allowed that to happen."

"Yeah," she agreed.

I noted to myself that she had just agreed that there was

a God and that she was indeed angry with him. That was progress.

"Claudia, being angry or offended when God doesn't do what we expect is natural, especially when we are in pain. The problem is that when you need him most, you have no access to him because you have pushed him away."

She opened her eyes wide with surprise at my statement, then softened and tilted her head to the side.

"If you are willing, I would like to help you release your anger toward God. I know that God really wants to hear how you feel," I said.

"He knows how I feel!" she snapped.

"Yes, he does," I said. "God can read your mind. He knows all your thoughts, but eavesdropping does not constitute a relationship."

She smiled at this.

I continued, "The basis of any good relationship is honesty. God wants to hear how you feel—and how you felt. Abandoned, fearful, whatever you felt, tell him. He has big shoulders; he can take it. If you pretend nothing is wrong and give him the silent treatment, you are the one missing out."

"What good could possibly come from it?" she said.

"Claudia, if I had kept you waiting for two hours in the waiting room, you would probably be offended. You would be expecting an explanation. If I didn't apologize and explain myself, you might even assume that I didn't care, right?"

"Yeah." She gave me a skeptical look, but allowed me to go on.

"Well, when God doesn't meet our expectations, we are offended and want an explanation. He doesn't usually answer the *why* questions. God expects us to set aside our offenses and trust him based on his character—not blind faith, but faith based on the things that he has already done for us and shown us about himself."

"Like what?" she asked.

"I bet you have some things that you know came from God that you didn't deserve. You do live in San Diego, with the best weather on the planet," I suggested.

"I have a great husband," she said. "I don't deserve him. All I do is make his life miserable."

"There you go. What else?"

"My job: I have a job, at a time when I know a lot of people are out of work. My daughter. I love my daughter," she said, almost smiling now.

"Let me tell you what I have seen," I said. "Many people suffer physical problems because of something that happened in their past, such as what happened to you. They are unable or unwilling to forgive someone who hurt them, and a couple of things happen. It drives them away from God, and it becomes a poison in their physical bodies that crops up as all sorts of problems."

She was listening intently now.

"Sometimes they have headaches, sometimes they can't sleep, and sometimes their immune systems get so compromised that diseases get the upper hand on them," I said.

"What do you do with people like that?" she asked.

"I recommend that they forgive anyone who hurt them, and I help them talk to God if they choose," I said. "Some people need to admit that they are angry with God. I would never push you into it, but I think telling God how badly these things hurt would do you good. Honesty is the basis of relationship. I recommend that you do it respectfully, but whatever you say, he can take it. He'd like you to tell him directly."

She waited a moment.

"I'm willing to try," she said.

"Okay. Why don't you start by telling God how you feel about what happened?" I said.

She paused long enough that I thought I'd lost her and that she would cut the appointment short. Then she said, "God, where were you when I was molested? Why did you let that happen?"

"Did you feel abandoned?" I prompted.

"I felt like you abandoned me, like you didn't care."

The sentiments hung in the air for a moment.

"Think about what else you are angry or frustrated about, and tell him that," I said.

"I'm angry with my mother," she said. "She has been so vindictive and controlling toward me. And my father has made such terrible choices. I hate to think that I'm even related to those people."

There was more silence.

"There are a number of things that have happened in your life that you don't understand," I said. "You are stuck waiting for an explanation before you trust God. You have already acknowledged that good things have happened to you that you didn't deserve. So you have questions about your past, but you seem to have evidence that God has been good to you."

"I guess so," she admitted with a half smile.

"If you are ready to move forward in your relationship with God, you will need to give up your demand to have an explanation for what happened to you. I am sure that you will get one someday, just not now."

Claudia thought carefully about what I was saying.

"I would like you to say something to God if you feel that it is the direction you want to move. Say, 'All these things that I don't understand I'm moving to the side, and God, you can explain them to me later. We have all eternity to talk about them. You don't need to explain them now, but I choose to believe that you are good and that you work all things for my good. You have my best interests in mind.'"[1]

By the time I finished saying this, she was weeping.

"God, I don't get it," she said, speaking now from the heart. "I don't know why this happened, but I will set my questions aside. You can explain them to me later. I choose to believe that you are good and that you have my best interests in mind, even if it doesn't feel like it."

She seemed to brighten and sit up straighter after she said this. Now that she was moving toward God, I asked if she was ready to forgive her mother and father. She said she was, and I helped her release that bitterness. She wept silently again, and my heart was gripped with sympathy to the point of pain.

Then she became quiet and still, with a peace she probably hadn't felt in years. I glanced at my office computer, which told me I was late. The next patient was waiting. Claudia looked up at me, then sat there for a moment taking her own measure.

"I feel very strange right now," she said. "Lighter, like a lot of stuff just left me."

"That's not unusual," I said. "You're on your way to a different, healthier life. I'm very impressed with what you've done today."

Late for my next appointment, I had to send her off with only my best wishes. I knew that bitterness was going to try to get back in, and I hadn't been able to offer Claudia anything positive to replace the bitterness that had resided in her heart. It would be easy for her to fall back into anger and bitterness the next time she spoke to her mother or father. Fortunately, I didn't have to wait long before I had the opportunity to follow up with her via phone.

"How are you doing?" I asked.

Her voice sounded cheerful and bubbly, no longer whiny.

"I'm doing so much better," she gushed. "Something happened to me in your office. I also found out that my mother-in-law has been praying for me. My husband has been telling me the same stuff you did, but I didn't believe it. Now people at work are asking me, 'What happened to you? Why are you so happy?'"

I had seen this many times before. People who wouldn't listen to relatives or religious leaders were open to reconnecting with God when encouraged by their doctors.

I gave her the name of a woman professional who could help her spiritually if she desired, and Claudia called her within the hour. She was moving toward spiritual restoration unusually quickly, from open disbelief to embracing God in the space of one visit. Her marriage began to improve, and she now looks at herself and her life with hope. It was as if the component parts of her faith had been lying around waiting for someone to help her put them together again.

• • •

Another patient, Jerry, had an enormous aneurysm pressing against his brain stem—a very dangerous situation. I had been called early one morning by the neurosurgical resident who had put him on the schedule for an emergency procedure. After seeing the CT scan remotely from my home computer, I agreed that it looked dangerous and should be fixed as soon as possible.

The aneurysm was located on the basilar artery in front of the brain stem, and it had grown so large—more than an inch in diameter—that it was compressing the brain stem, causing him trouble when he walked. Most aneurysms are less than 7 millimeters in diameter, about a quarter inch. Jerry's aneurysm was more than 25 millimeters (an inch), which boosted it into the giant category. All parts of the brain are surprisingly forgiving; they tend to accommodate an aneurysm or a tumor as long as it grows slowly. However, the brain stem, like the spinal cord with its tightly packed nerves, is affected earlier than other parts of the brain, and this aneurysm was now encroaching on the brain's territory. It was a situation that could soon prove fatal.

My first questions when confronting any case, even one this dangerous, are always, "Should we do something or should we do nothing? Is the best option to leave this alone? It has lasted this many years—what are the chances of its harming him now? Can we treat his symptoms without doing anything to the aneurysm?" I pondered these questions as I drove to the hospital that morning, but only after I arrived and saw more-detailed scans was I able to settle on a recommendation. The scans showed that the problem was even more serious than I had thought. The risk of stroke during or after surgery would be 25 percent or higher, but if we did nothing, he was likely to progress into debilitation and eventually death.

I went into the exam room and met Jerry, the "owner" of this aneurysm, for the first time. He was a short man of about sixty-five who looked as if he could survive in the jungle with nothing but a knife. I knew from talking to the neurosurgery resident that he was strongly independent and had waited as long as he could before considering treatment. Realizing that his symptoms were only getting worse and that he would soon be wheelchair-bound, he grudgingly agreed to look at his medical options.

I began interviewing him before the procedure.

"What do you do for a living?" I asked, trying to learn

about him and the context in which he was coming in for surgery.

"Retired," he said.

"What was your career?" I asked. He looked unwilling to answer.

"Odd jobs here and there," he said, and gave no further explanation.

"Tell me about your symptoms," I said. He began to explain in clipped sentences that he had been getting slowly weaker on his right side. He was still able to get around town on the bus system, but he had started walking with a limp.

"Do you have anyone who can drive you where you need to go?" I asked.

"I live alone," he said.

"No friends or neighbors?"

"Not really," he said.

Either he was a true loner or he was just bluffing because he was scared. In any case, I was learning that he wasn't the kind of man who liked divulging information or depending on others.

"Well, it looks as though the problem is getting worse," I said. "This procedure is risky, but if we do nothing, your symptoms will probably continue and you will eventually become incapacitated."

"I get that, Doc," he said. "It's why I'm here."

Something about his manner struck me as odd. He was treating our time together as if it were a routine visit to the dentist, and he was about to get a filling. I wondered whether he was taking the risks of the procedure seriously. I decided to change direction with my questions.

"Did anyone come with you today?" I asked.

"No," he said.

"Any family in town that you could call?"

"No."

"The reason I ask is that this is a high-risk procedure."

"How high risk?"

"Very high," I responded. "You have a giant aneurysm next to the most important part of your brain. The vessel has taken on an unusual shape and will be difficult to repair, if it can be repaired at all. It could be fatal. I think you have at least a one in four chance of having a major stroke or dying."

A startled look passed over his face.

"Are you serious?" he asked.

"I am," I said.

He did not seem emotionally prepared to hear this, and I wondered why he thought the risk would be low. After all, it was a giant aneurysm and he was already becoming paralyzed.

"I haven't heard anything about dying," he said.

I was sorry that this was the first time he was hearing it, and I said so. "This is a very risky procedure," I repeated.

Jerry looked down at the ground and grimaced. It was painfully apparent that this was new information to him and that he had never really thought about dying. He began to breathe heavily and make small gestures of frustration and distress, as if being rushed into a situation he hadn't expected.

His sentences got longer, too.

"I need to call my wife," he said. "Actually, she's my ex-wife, but she's the most important person in my life besides my son."

"Sure, go ahead. You can call her from here," I said, and he took out his cell phone and dialed.

In the space of time this afforded me, I thought about what else I might do to fill in the gaps for Jerry, now that I realized he had not been made fully aware of the risks involved with such a procedure. He should have had time to consider the implications, and ideally he should have had a group of supportive people with him to comfort and encourage him before and after the surgery. Instead, here he was—alone, in clear emotional distress, and completely unready for something of this magnitude.

He reached his ex-wife's voice mail. As soon as he heard the recording of her voice, this previously impassive man began weeping and was unable to stop. Finally, when it was time to leave a message, he squeaked out the words, "This is Jerry. They're going to do a procedure, and I might not survive."

He hung up, tried to compose himself, then dialed his son but failed to reach him as well. He put down the phone and choked back tears. He looked anguished. In the meantime I handed him a tissue and began studying another bit of information in his chart that must have been seen as inconsequential in light of his aneurysm. His blood work from the morning had just returned and the numbers were noticeably low.

"Your blood count came back low this morning. Do you have any idea where you might be losing blood?" I asked.

"Angiomas," he said, his tears subsiding a bit. "All over the inside of my gut. They bleed."

"How often?"

"Once a week."

"How much blood do you lose?" I asked.

"About a pint."

"You lose a pint of blood each week?"

"Yeah," he said.

Angiomas are small bumps that look like red moles. They are a rare cause of bleeding anywhere along the gastro-intestinal tract. Jerry was describing spontaneous hemorrhag-ing that was causing a significant loss of blood—a fact that had major implications for his surgery.

"Have you had them taken care of?" I asked.

He shook his head. "I don't like hospitals," he said.

This was a problem. I would have to use blood thinners during his procedure and throughout his recovery to lessen the risk of clotting and stroke, but if one of those angiomas popped, Jerry might bleed uncontrollably. I calculated the risk for bleeding to death after the surgery at 50 percent if we put him on blood thinners as planned.

"Jerry, let's take stock of where we are," I said. "This aneu-rysm is pressing on your brain stem. You are losing the use of your right side and can no longer walk without a cane. We were planning to do the surgery today, but your bleeding problem needs to be looked at—perhaps we can help that today. You seem to be learning just now about how risky the surgery is, so I think we should delay it. But I have an idea. Why don't we do an angiogram today and look at your aneurysm as well as the bleeding sites in your intestines? An angiogram would tell me a lot more about the blood flow in the aneurysm. I will also have a radiologist help me embolize, or plug up, any bleeding sites in your intestines. If we can stop you from bleeding from the angiomas, the treatment of the aneurysm will be much safer."

"Okay," he said, a bit relieved.

"I recommend we do that today and not treat the aneurysm yet."

He nodded. This seemed to be an acceptable pathway for both of us.

"Jerry, every procedure, even an angiogram, has a risk. I typically pray with my patients before procedures, and I'd like to do that now," I said. "Is that all right with you?"

He looked surprised, but he consented. I placed my hand on his shoulder. He stared straight ahead.

"God, you know all about Jerry," I prayed. "I ask you for safety today during this procedure. Amen."

I looked up. Jerry was still staring straight ahead as if nothing had happened, as if he were biding his time waiting for me to tie my shoe.

The anesthesiologist was waiting outside the exam room. Jerry was taken to the procedure room and sedated. Scrubbed and ready, I soon stood at his side and put the catheter up through his femoral artery. I injected dye and took a high-resolution angiogram, which gave me a virtual video of the vessels near his aneurysm. It was big and ugly. There was no easy way to fix it.

After the angiogram, we spent several hours identifying and trying to plug the arteries that were feeding the angiomas in his intestines. We thought we had achieved a result that would prevent him from bleeding. I went to visit with him in the recovery room.

"How do you feel?" I asked.

"Fine," he said.

"The procedure went well," I said as I showed him the images. "I got a good look at your aneurysm."

He nodded. "Thank you," he said. I planned to delay the next procedure two weeks, and I wanted to get him thinking about fundamental things, to be prepared for it emotionally, psychologically, and spiritually.

"We talked earlier about the risk of death. With your two conditions, death is a significant possibility with or without this procedure," I said. "Where are you on your spiritual journey? Have you thought about that at all?"

"Nah," he said, "I can't believe in God."

"Why?" I asked gently.

"I've seen too much," he said with contempt.

My silence invited more explanation.

"I've traveled around and seen too much to believe anything," he repeated.

"Okay," I said. "Some people like to settle their accounts before going into something like this."

He nodded unenthusiastically to let me know he'd heard me. It was clear that more probing in this area would be unfruitful and perhaps even harmful.

"Then I'll see you in a week or so," I said. "If you have any questions, feel free to call me. Rest up. You're doing great."

"Thank you," he said.

The next week Jerry had another bleeding episode from his GI tract, which earned him a trip to the emergency room. The ER said he had lost a pint of blood and was anemic. He still wanted to move forward with the procedure, to try to preserve his ability to walk independently, and two weeks later he was in the pre-op area again. His son and a couple of neighbors from his apartment complex were in the waiting room. They did not seem to know each other, and an uncomfortable silence engulfed them.

I went to visit Jerry in pre-op and found him slightly chattier this time. I arrived early, allowing time to talk, in case he'd had a change of heart and wanted to open up. We greeted each other, and I went through my pre-op checklist to make sure he fully understood the high risks of what we were trying to do and what might happen if we failed. Then I again addressed his spiritual life.

"Jerry, I know you said last time that spiritual things aren't very important to you, but I make a habit of asking patients if there is anything they need to do to make peace with God before a procedure like this," I said. "It could be something you feel unsettled about, or need forgiveness for, or something that would give you peace going into surgery."

He sighed. "I really don't believe in that stuff," he said. He went quiet for a moment, but instead of clamming up completely, he continued talking. "I saw so many starving kids in Africa," he said. "Dying kids. I never figured out how God could let them suffer that way. They never did anything to deserve it."

"Why were you in Africa?" I asked curiously.

"Work," he answered cryptically.

"What kind of work?"

"Just work," he parried—then he finally relented, looking at the ground. "I was a mercenary, paramilitary. Did for-hire stuff. Various places. Different groups."

I nodded and received the information carefully.

"Sounds like interesting work. Which African countries were you in?"

"Whichever ones needed a war started," he said grimly and with a slight chuckle. "These governments—they were so corrupt. You almost didn't feel bad, taking out these guys. I should probably be dead myself. All my friends died—of bullets and land mines. I'm not sure why I escaped. I haven't been able to figure that out."

I kept listening, giving him the respect of my silence.

"We trained rebel groups," he elaborated. "Brought in weapons, got rid of bad guys."

"Dangerous?"

"Real dangerous. But the work wasn't what bothered me," he said. "It was the inhumanity of the people I worked with. It sounds stupid, but sometimes when we were on the boats, other guys—mercenaries from other countries—would shoot the crocodiles on the banks. How could they shoot innocent animals like that? They just played target practice with 'em. And the children—everywhere we went, I saw them suffer for nothing."

I nodded. "Have any close calls?" I asked. "Plenty," he said. "We were ambushed on our boat. Ambushed in buildings. Couple of times I thought I would never make it out alive. In fact, one time I was the only one who did make it out alive. Everyone I worked with eventually got killed. I'm the only one left."

"So why did you do it?"

"Good money. Very good money. Exciting work. Camaraderie."

"So the reason you can't believe in God is because of what you saw and what you did?" I asked a little more boldly.

He exhaled. "A little of both," he said. "I wouldn't have done what I did if I didn't think the governments were unjust. But you can't justify everything. Some of the guys I served with were heartless. After a while I was afraid I was becoming like them. And I hated seeing the starving kids."

"I wonder if you've ever told God how unfair it was, all the things you saw."

"He doesn't need me to tell him," he said.

"Not for his sake, but for yours," I said. "It seems that you haven't made sense of it."

He thought a moment.

"Maybe so," he replied. "I still feel angry about it."

"God is not afraid of your anger," I said. "He can take whatever you throw at him as long as you are honest. Making peace with God starts by being honest. Are you interested in telling him some of these things?"

"All right," he said. "Can't hurt."

I sat in a chair next to his bed. "God," I said to start him off, "Jerry has seen a lot of suffering in his life. He'd like to talk to you about that today."

On cue, after my brief silence, Jerry began to speak.

"I don't know why I saw so much suffering and unfairness," he said. "There were innocent children dying. Inhumane behavior on both sides. Cruelty. Why would you let those things happen? How could you just stand by and watch?"

He stopped for a moment, then opened his eyes, startled, as if receiving a revelation. Then he continued as if speaking to himself.

"I guess people did those things to other people," he said. "Maybe the suffering wasn't God's fault. God gives men free will. It was . . . people."

I nodded. "One of the things I tell patients is that they don't have to understand why things happen in order to trust God," I said. "If you want, you can set those things aside and trust him now, even though you don't have all the answers. It sounds as though you are getting some new insights just by talking to him."

He nodded, and I continued.

"One of the best ways to further the conversation between you and God is to mention some of the things you're thankful for," I suggested. "Can you think of anything that falls in that category?"

"Yeah."

"Do you want to take a moment and thank him?"

"Sure." He closed his eyes and put his head down. "Thank you for all the times my life was spared," he said. "You brought me home every time. My friends are all . . . gone. Thank you that the bullets and the land mines and machetes never got me. Somehow I made it. I feel like you deserve credit for that."

He was quiet.

"Jerry, is there anything you need to be forgiven for?" I asked.

"Yeah," he said as he nodded slowly. "Lots."

He thought a moment, and I gave him time.

"I know I should do this," he said after a while. "God, forgive me for . . . the things I've done that weren't right. You know what I did that was wrong. Forgive me so those things don't weigh on my mind anymore."

He was quiet.

"Feel better?" I asked.

"Yeah," he said. He seemed more human than I had ever seen him, less the aged warrior and more a tender man facing the end of life alone. I shook his hand.

"Any more questions for me?" I asked.

"No, Doc, I think I'm ready," he said and smiled. I left to prepare for his procedure.

The surgery was difficult. I couldn't use a stent as I had

hoped because that would have required Jerry to be on a blood thinner regimen for six weeks. That would risk a fatal bleed from the angiomas in his bowel. Instead, I used a small balloon to hold open the vessel while I placed coil after coil in the mega-aneurysm. The procedure was successful, but the day following the surgery, he suffered a stroke and had difficulty speaking. His son was there to comfort him. His neighbors lingered in the waiting room out of obligation, but none of them seemed to know him well enough to offer any real encouragement. Whatever community he had known in the mercenary trade was gone. His social network was too thin to offer support in his moment of crisis.

Jerry was understandably angry about his loss of function. The surgery had extended his life, but at the expense of his independence. With rehabilitation he recovered some of his ability to talk, but he was as terse after surgery as he had been before. When I asked if he was making any progress on his spiritual journey, he said, "No." We never again spoke at length about spiritual things. My prayer and hope was that he continued talking to God about the pain from his past and the frustrations he had as he fought this new battle—but for me, that's where the story ended.

• • •

Then there was Betty, a thin, eighty-seven-year-old woman with a lively manner. I met her as she was waiting nervously for me in the exam room. She had been referred to me after tripping over a curb and falling while carrying her bridge club newsletter to the post office. The resulting bump on her head prompted her doctor to request a CT scan. It showed a brain aneurysm that had nothing to do with her fall and that was not very serious.

My conversation with Betty was quick and conclusive: the aneurysm had never bled or caused her a problem. She was already in her late eighties. To fix it surgically risked causing a stroke, and that was, in my opinion, riskier than doing nothing. I recommended leaving it alone. She agreed, and we found ourselves finished with the substance of her appointment. Because it had gone so fast, I felt obligated to give her a little more value for her time. She was still wringing her hands and didn't seem in a hurry to leave.

"You seem anxious," I offered. "When people are in their eighties, I always recommend that they consider end-of-life issues before there are any surprises. Were you raised with a faith or religion?"

She had been listening pleasantly, but when I mentioned religion she gave me a sideways look.

"Methodist," she said, "but I don't believe in anything now. Why did you ask me that?"

"I like to know where people are coming from and what is important to them," I said. "Some people say faith helps them cope with the challenges that can arise in later life. At eighty-seven, even though I'm sure you have many years left, it's good to make sure you are at peace with dying."

She shrugged her shoulders. "I'm at peace. When you die, then you're dead. That's all there is to it."

I didn't say anything immediately, but just nodded. She went on.

"At my age I go to a lot of funerals and hate it when they talk about religious themes or an afterlife," she said. "They should keep the discussion strictly to the person's life. I don't like being preached to."

"So nothing worries you about the end of life?" I asked.

"The only thing that worries me is that people will find my house in a mess after I'm gone and think I was an untidy, disorganized person who did not finish the projects she started," she said.

She gave a firm nod to punctuate the sentence.

"It sounds like you've thought this through," I said.

"Of course I have," she responded. "My ex-husband and my husband died the same week, one year apart. A dozen people close to me have died in the last five years. I'm well acquainted with death."

"I'll just ask, then, is there anything unresolved in your life you'd like to take care of?" I asked.

"Aside from my messy house? No," she said.

"Once you're dead, will you really care what people think about you or your housekeeping?" I asked. "You can probably keep your house as messy as you want."

"True," she said, reflecting for a moment. "I guess you're right about that."

"Is there anything else bothering you?" I asked.

She fell quiet.

Finally, she opened up. "I haven't spoken of this to anyone, but there is a painful family situation," she said. After hesitating, she continued. "My son wanted to marry a woman, but I wasn't for it and put pressure on him to leave her. She told him that she was pregnant, and he committed suicide. Now she is suing our family for his money. She says it's for the child. Most of the money has already gone to lawyers."

"I am sorry to hear that," I said. "That sounds very difficult."

"I haven't told anyone about my son, even when I hear my friends sharing stories about their family problems," she said. "I'm just too embarrassed. If they found out, they would know that my life isn't what it seems to be. The worst of it is, I can't see my two-year-old grandchild because of the lawsuit."

"Are you angry at your son for killing himself?" I asked.

"Not really," she said. This surprised me.

"Are you angry at God for allowing it to happen?" I asked.

"No," she said.

It was curious to me that her opinions were so firm, even in the face of such pain and trouble. My spiritual questions were not resonating with her. *Can she not see God wanting to help her with her grief over these losses?* I wondered. Then something unusual happened: I felt a strange prompting to compliment her. I prayed, *God, show me the beauty you see in her.* Immediately I began to see the things God saw when he looked at Betty. Not her faults, but her strengths. Not her failures, but her successes. Not her timidity, but her courage.

Not her lack of faith, but the fact that she simply had not yet recognized God's goodness in her life.

"You know, I am really impressed with you; you are an amazing woman," I said. "You were carrying your bridge club newsletter to the post office when you fell and hit your head. You invested a lot of time and effort to put that together to bless your friends. You obviously want good communication and good relationships with your loved ones. I find that really commendable. You didn't have to do it, and nobody paid you to do it. You did it because you have a big and beautiful heart."

She stared at me. Then her eyes welled up and she started crying. Her face turned red with emotion. I handed her a tissue.

"I can tell that you love to laugh and that you enjoy making others happy," I continued. "You are an intelligent woman who has kept herself in good mental and physical health for eighty-seven years. I see such strong character in you."

She sat crying for a moment.

"Well, thank you. I don't know what to say to all that," she said, blowing her nose.

"When you've lived life like you have, you could really use your experiences and wisdom to encourage others," I said. "You have made it through some tough times, and now you have the opportunity to help others who are on the same journey. I don't think you need to be ashamed about your family situation. You might share your son's story and allow others to gain strength from your experience and to support you. I think what you've been through has added to your character."

She smiled at me through glistening eyes. I was speaking the truth as I saw it from God's perspective, and her response told me that nobody had told her such things in a long time—if ever.

"I think I might just do that," she said.

I was hesitant to ask to pray for her, but decided to test the waters. I did not want to miss an opportunity to bless this beautiful woman.

"I have another patient to see, but I would love to pray a blessing over you before you go," I said. "Would that be okay?"

"Oh, yes," she said enthusiastically and grabbed both of my hands, holding them tightly while bowing her head.

"God, thank you for Betty," I said. "I know you are proud of her. You love the way she cares for her family and friends. You love it when she laughs. You love her mind and how well she has taken care of herself all these years. I ask you to bless her relationships and her health. In Jesus' name, Amen."

She stood.

"I have to hug you," she said and flung her arms around me. I was surprised, given how seemingly self-sufficient and resistant to faith she had been. As we entered the hallway and walked to the nurses' station, she put her arm through mine and clung to me as if I were her date to the prom. At the desk I offered her one of my cards.

"I enjoyed talking with you," I said. "Have a great day."

But she just stood there with me and the nurses. She

didn't want to leave. For a few moments she basked in something that she perhaps hadn't felt in a long time—love and appreciation for all that she was. When she finally left, I was expecting not to see her again.

Six months later she appeared on my schedule again, but I did not recognize who it was until I went into the exam room. Then I recalled her face and our earlier visit.

"Betty, how are you?" I asked, shaking her hand.

She beamed. "Just fine," she said. "I wanted to discuss my aneurysm again." I think we both knew she didn't need a visit for such a nonthreatening aneurysm, but I sat down and reviewed the old scan to see if my opinion was still the same. It was, and I confirmed that her aneurysm was just the same as I remembered it. Nothing needed to be done.

"We talked about fixing it last time, but because of your age, the risks were higher than the benefits," I said.

She nodded and then started talking.

"When I called to make an appointment awhile ago, I was told you were on a medical trip helping the poor," she said. "I have some friends who spend their time doing things for the poor and homeless downtown. I'm not as good as those people—I spend most of my time playing bridge, which is selfish, I guess. But I was thinking that maybe I should help them sometime. I have time to do good things for the poor, too."

"That sounds like something you would enjoy," I said.

"I think I would," she agreed. "You know, I just wanted to tell you that I'm exploring new things in my life."

Her eyes met mine and conveyed the importance of these words.

"That's very encouraging," I said. "I am really pleased that you want to help the poor. I think you are moving in the right direction."

She beamed, receiving the compliment. With that, having accomplished her purpose for the visit, she stood and I walked her to the nurses' station. She hugged me and went out happily.

As a doctor or health-care provider, it can be easy to focus only on people's problems. Obviously that is why they are in the office. But there is more to medicine than fixing problems—there are healing words. By telling Betty what I saw in her, I helped her to realize that there was a purpose to her life beyond playing cards. There is great power in affirming people's good qualities—their inner beauty, kindness, strength, and love. My interaction with Betty taught me that affirmation may be God's favorite way to move people toward their destinies. After all, it is God's kindness that draws us to himself.

In his kindness he drew me. With the particular set of skills he gave me, he allows me the profound privilege of having a hand in physical healing—and sometimes, even more incredibly, of helping my patients find their way to emotional or spiritual health. It is a privilege that humbles me and for which I am grateful to God with every new patient I meet.

Epilogue

ANNETTE, THE LITTLE GIRL who had narrowly survived the surgery to block off her large DAVF a year earlier, was back on the operating table—and about to die. I watched helplessly as her vital signs plummeted. Dr. Thompson and I looked at each other in powerless frustration—what had gone wrong? Why was her body suddenly shutting down after what had been a successful surgery?

I wondered what I would tell Annette's parents now, after all we had been through together. How could I let them know that their long journey was ending this way, with a lifeless girl on an operating table? How could I even face them?

As I watched her numbers drop on the monitor, there was

nothing I could do but prepare to perform CPR when her heart stopped. Maybe we could keep her circulation going long enough to figure out what had gone wrong.

● ● ●

Annette had made dramatic improvements after her previous surgery. She had learned to walk using a walker and had even taken twenty steps on her own. Her speech had come back much better than expected.

However, her DAVF was one of the largest and most aggressive that I had ever seen. Within a year it had re-formed both above and below the glue injection, building new connections around the blocked vessels. I had never dealt with anything quite like this. I felt as if I were playing a game of chess with Annette's body: for every move I made, it made a countermove.

Dural AVFs in children are especially difficult to shut down because children's bodies are full of growth hormones, which cause the DAVF to regrow quickly by recruiting nearby arteries. The new growth of the DAVF necessitated another surgery to try to block it off again, but this time I couldn't go up through the affected vessel because I had blocked it off with glue the previous time. I would have to go through the skull.

My plan was to close off the entire network of veins in that part of the brain in two stages: First, I would block the jugular vein in the neck, depriving the DAVF of any outflow.

Then, in an open procedure, I would expose the problem vein in the brain, put a clamp on it upstream from the DAVF connections, and inject glue to close off the whole area down to the jugular. The only way to stop the rogue arteries from making connections to that vein would be to seal off the outflow, forcing the blood to go elsewhere. It was such a complex pediatric procedure that I needed to work in conjunction with a specialized neurosurgeon, Dr. Thompson.

The risks were manifold. I would be permanently blocking one of Annette's two jugular veins, which are responsible for draining blood from the head. You never know what might happen when you close a jugular, though I was rather certain that the other side could handle the extra outflow. Jugular veins are like kidneys: you'd rather have two, but you can live with just one. Nevertheless, it was a testament to how serious her DAVF problem was that we would perform such drastic destructive procedures to stop its progression.

After that, we would drill open a section of skull right over the troubled vein. Opening the skull invites all sorts of problems, from infection to problems involving the spinal fluid. I would inject glue directly into the vein, but because we were in a neurosurgical operating room, it would be much more difficult to see what was happening. The quality of the mobile X-ray machines we use in operating rooms is nowhere near as high as those in the radiology department, where most endovascular brain procedures are performed. There was no way to bring the better machine into the operating room because it was fixed in position in its procedure room. Furthermore, there was no way to do the surgery in the radiology department because it was not designed to handle open surgery.

All this meant that Annette's procedure would be anything but routine.

• • •

On the day of surgery I prayed with Annette's parents as they held her. By that time I had no inhibitions about inviting God into the medical process. In the operating room, the first step of the procedure went well. I closed the jugular with a device that is basically a high-tech metal cork. It stuck firmly in the vessel, immediately shutting off the flow in the jugular vein. Annette's body responded perfectly: the blood from her head simply flowed down the other jugular, but did not overwhelm it.

Then we began the open surgery, removing the bone behind Annette's ear with a burr drill. In some cases we might have cut out a section of skull, kept it in a sterile towel during the procedure, then replaced it when we were finished. However, in this case we essentially sanded the bone away with a motorized hand drill to create a hole one inch by two inches right over the vein. Once this was accomplished, a clip was placed across the vein. Now this vein was sealed shut between the clip in the head and the cork farther down the jugular in the neck, creating a closed area. It had no outflow or inflow, except where the AVM vessels had connected to it.

Standing near Annette's head, I could not see her face, just the opening in the skull behind her ear. I was looking at the dura mater, the brain's cover. The large vein that I was looking for coursed just underneath. I felt the stress of the moment. We were at the most significant point in the surgery, and it had taken us four hours to get there.

Through the hole in the skull I threaded an intravenous catheter into the vein. Blood spurted out, indicating that the vessels had not yet clotted off but were still patent, or open. I injected glue with a syringe. One second . . . two seconds . . . three seconds. I wanted to block all possible connections and fill the entire vein. When I finished the injection and pulled out the needle, no blood came back, which meant that the flow was cut off.

Before backing away and letting Dr. Thompson and the neurosurgery resident close up, I noticed that there was a second venous pouch behind Annette's ear, separate from this vein and just under the skin. I injected this pouch with glue and let it harden. Then I stepped away from the table to allow them to close up the skull. At the back table I put the needles in the sharps container and removed my gloves. My part of the procedure was over.

Then, suddenly, Annette's condition began to deteriorate. Rapidly.

The first one to notice was the anesthesiologist. He was sitting next to his cart, which had flat-panel monitors showing indicators such as blood pressure, heart rate, and oxygen saturation.

"Any reason her blood pressure is dropping?" asked the anesthesiologist loudly from his position on the other side of Annette. "You guys doing something up there?"

"No," said Dr. Thompson.

"Heart rate's dropping too," said the anesthesiologist.

Suddenly the alarms on his monitors began going off. Annette's blood pressure, which had been at 130, was now at 100—and falling fast. Her heart rate was also dropping. And her temperature was rising. Something very serious was happening but none of us knew what.

The anesthesiologist sprang into action. Normally, anesthesiologists are the wallflowers in the operating room, staying quiet behind their protective blue drape. But with Annette's vitals dropping, it was his duty to try to stabilize her quickly.

"I need a blood-gas reading," he said to the tech while drawing blood into tubes from the port in Annette's femoral artery. "Get me STAT labs on these!"

The tech rushed the tubes to the lab. The anesthesiologist was already searching the drawers of his cart for glass vials of drugs and injecting their contents into the IV drip to try to get Annette's blood pressure to stabilize. Her blood pressure continued downward.

. . . 90 . . . 80 . . . 70 . . .

"God, what is happening?" I prayed under my breath. "What's gone wrong?"

The fact that all of Annette's vital signs were falling at once was ominous. It meant that major systems had been affected—but by what? To have your heart rate and blood pressure drop at the same time indicates a severe and unusual problem. Usually if the blood pressure goes down, the heart rate goes up to compensate, but with both going down simultaneously, it might be neurological. Had the glue found its way to the brain stem? The possibility made me shudder.

There might be other possibilities as well. There might have been an air embolus—a bubble of air that is sucked into an open vein from the outside. This is rare, but it can be fatal if the bubble travels to the lungs. Or the problem might be her breathing tube. The anesthesiologist, who was responsible for the endotracheal tube, listened to the lung sounds to see if the tube had become displaced. The tube was in its proper place. And Annette was getting worse.

The uncertainty was so agonizing that for a moment I had to stop watching the vital signs drop on the monitor. I knew there was nothing more I could do but pray. I turned away and began begging God to intervene. Facing the wall, I implored desperately, "God, you've got to help her. Don't let her die now. Please, we need your help. There's nothing we can do."

Nearby, Dr. Thompson and the neurosurgery resident were in limbo. Just before Annette's condition changed, they had been putting a calcium paste into the opening of her head to refabricate the skull. Now everyone was frozen in place thinking, as I was, that in a minute Annette would go into cardiac arrest and we would have to start pumping on her chest to try to keep her alive. A three-year-old doesn't have many reserves. Something had to stop her free fall.

The sickness in my heart grew to a throbbing mass. I couldn't imagine going out to the waiting room to tell the family, friends of mine by now, that we had come all this way to have Annette die on the operating table. The only consolation I had was that God would be with me, no matter what happened.

The anesthesiologist was still barking orders to the nurses and the other tech. Dr. Thompson and I looked across the room at each other, helpless. The alarms beat a menacing rhythm to the unfolding scene. Eventually, the anesthesiologist reached over and slapped them off. Now we stared at the monitors and watched the numbers fall in eerie silence.

The anesthesiologist yanked open drawers and searched for more vials, glass clinking against glass like wind chimes. Finding the one he wanted, he turned it upside down, pushed in a syringe, and jammed the needle into the rubber port on the IV drip. This medicine would kick-start the heart, stimulating it to pump harder and thus cause the blood pressure to increase. He also opened up the IV lines to put more fluid into Annette's system, none of which would help if Annette's system was shutting down.

. . . 60 . . . 50 . . . 40 . . .

I began preparing myself to perform CPR. Then, just as I was about to step toward the table, the numbers stopped dropping. We all stared at the monitors.

. . . 40 . . . 40 . . . 40 . . .

"Stabilizing," the anesthesiologist said after a moment. I couldn't immediately believe it.

"Pressure's increasing," the anesthesiologist said, checking another indicator. Then the number moved again, but this time in the right direction.

. . . 40 . . . 50 . . . 50 . . . 50 . . . 60 . . .

Everyone breathed again. The anesthesiologist exhaled audibly. For two full minutes we watched as Annette's vitals crept upward, indicating that whatever the crisis had been, it had passed—at least for the moment.

Dr. Thompson and the neurosurgery resident stepped forward and began to resume the work of closing the skull. We didn't know what had happened, but they knew, as we all did, that we needed to get Annette off the table before it happened again.

"God, thank you," I prayed silently with deep emotion. "Thank you."

I continued to breathe thanks as I waited and watched. Thirty minutes later they finished applying the calcium putty to the hole in Annette's skull and sewed the skin over it. Now we would wait for her to wake up.

She woke up so slowly that we began to worry that she had suffered brain damage. It took an hour before the nurses informed me she was moving her arms and legs, and for the first time that day I felt relief. I went out and talked to her parents.

"We had a scare, and we aren't sure why," I told them, "but the fact that she is moving her limbs means that the glue did not go to the brain stem, which is reason to be very thankful. We might never know exactly what happened, given the complexity of the procedure, but she seems to be okay now."

They sighed, hugged each other, and grasped my hand.

Annette remained in the hospital for two days, then went home and picked up right where she had left off. She started walking again with her walker. She resumed speech therapy. In spite of the scare, our procedure had been a success. I hoped that it was the last one she would ever need.

• • •

Neurosurgery, like life itself, is full of surprises. No surgeon, not even the most highly trained, can save a life alone. During this dramatic procedure I was reminded that the outcomes of procedures, and of our very lives, are ultimately in God's hands. He wants to be involved in the details of everything we do, no matter our position or profession. My practice and my life have been transformed because I have learned to pray with my patients. In the beginning the risk seemed high, but it was meager compared to the gain. I have learned firsthand that, as radiant sunlight melts away fog, God infuses life-giving hope into the darkest circumstances. If we look for him, we will find him,[1] and the journey will be amazing.

Notes

CHAPTER 1

1. Curlin FA et al., "Physicians' Observations and Interpretations of the Influence of Religion and Spirituality on Health," *Arch Intern Med* (2007) 167:(7)649–54.

2. Magyar-Russell G et al., "Ophthalmology Patients' Religious and Spiritual Beliefs," *Arch Ophthalmol* (2008) 126(9):1262–65.

3. Drawn from the following articles:

   Carson JW et al., "Forgiveness and Chronic Low Back Pain: A Preliminary Study Examining the Relationship of Forgiveness to Pain, Anger, and Psychological Distress," *J Pain* (2005 Feb) 6(2):84–91.

   Dezutter J et al., "God, Image, and Happiness in Chronic Pain Patients: The Mediating Role of Disease Interpretation," *Pain Med* (2010 May) 11(5):765–73.

   Chronic pain patients with positive God images had greater levels of happiness. One's emotional experience of God has an influence on happiness.

Friedberg JP et al., "Relationship between Forgiveness and Psychological and Physiological Indices in Cardiac Patients," *Int J Behav Med* (2009) 16(3):205–11.
Stress, anxiety, depression, and cholesterol were all improved by forgiveness.
Hansen MJ et al., "A Palliative Care Intervention in Forgiveness Therapy for Elderly Terminally Ill Cancer Patients," *J Palliative Care* (2009 Spring) 25(1):51–60.
Hope and quality of life significantly improved in cancer patients who learned forgiveness.
Lawler KA et al., "A Change of Heart: Cardiovascular Correlates of Forgiveness in Response to Interpersonal Conflict," *J Behav Med* (2003 Oct) 26(5):373–93.
Lawler KA et al., "The Unique Effects of Forgiveness on Health: An Exploration of Pathways," *J Behav Med* (2005 Apr) 28(2):157–67.
Webb JR et al., "Forgiveness and Health-Related Outcomes among People with Spinal Cord Injury," *Disability and Rehabilitation* (2010) 32(5):360–66.
Spinal cord injury patients who forgive others reported significantly higher health status.
Whited MC et al., "The Influence of Forgiveness and Apology on Cardiovascular Reactivity and Recovery in Response to Mental Stress," *J Behav Med* (2010 Aug) 33(4):293–304.
Forgiveness positively affects cardiac recovery from stressful events.
Worthington EL et al., "Forgiveness, Health, and Well-Being: A Review of Evidence for Emotional Versus Decisional Forgiveness, Dispositional Forgivingness, and Reduced Unforgiveness," *J Behav Med* (2007 Aug) 30(4):291–302.

CHAPTER 2
1. MacLean CD et al., "Patient Preference for Physician Discussion and Practice of Spirituality," *J Gen Intern Med* (2003 Jan) 18(1):38–43.
2. King DE, Bushwick B, "Beliefs and Attitudes of Hospital Inpatients about Faith Healing and Prayer," *J Fam Pract* (1994 Oct) 39 (4):349–52.
3. Maugans TA, Wadland WC, "Religion and Family Medicine: A Survey of Physicians and Patients," *J Fam Pract* (1991 Feb) 32(2):210–13.
4. Matthews DA et al., Religious Commitment and Health Status: A Review of the Research and Implications for Family Medicine," *Arch Fam Med* (1998 Mar-Apr) 7(2):118–24.
5. Larimore WL et al., "Should Clinicians Incorporate Positive Spirituality

into Their Practices? What Does the Evidence Say?" *Ann Behav Med* (2002 Winter) 24(1):69–73.

CHAPTER 3

1. I cannot remember everything I said to Joan after she experienced the "cloudlike" feeling. What I have included here is what I typically would say to someone who wanted to move toward God.

CHAPTER 4

1. Letter reproduced with the permission of "Dr. Willard," whose name has been changed.

CHAPTER 5

1. Samuel brought all the tribes of Israel before the LORD, and the tribe of Benjamin was chosen by lot. Then he brought each family of the tribe of Benjamin before the LORD, and the family of the Matrites was chosen. And finally Saul son of Kish was chosen from among them. But when they looked for him, he had disappeared! So they asked the LORD, "Where is he?" And the LORD replied, "He is hiding among the baggage." So they found him and brought him out, and he stood head and shoulders above anyone else. Then Samuel said to all the people, "This is the man the LORD has chosen as your king. No one in all Israel is like him!" And all the people shouted, "Long live the king!" (1 Samuel 10:20-24).

CHAPTER 7

1. A cheerful heart is good medicine, but a broken spirit saps a person's strength (Proverbs 17:22).

2. If you forgive those who sin against you, your heavenly Father will forgive you. But if you refuse to forgive others, your Father will not forgive your sins (Matthew 6:14-15).

3. If we confess our sins to him, he is faithful and just to forgive us our sins and to cleanse us from all wickedness (1 John 1:9).

4. Confess your sins to each other and pray for each other so that you may be healed. The earnest prayer of a righteous person has great power and produces wonderful results (James 5:16).

CHAPTER 8

1. If you forgive those who sin against you, your heavenly Father will forgive you. But if you refuse to forgive others, your Father will not forgive your sins (Matthew 6:14-15).

CHAPTER 10

1. The details of this story and these remarks were printed with the permission of "Charlotte," whose name has been changed.

CHAPTER 12

1. We know that God causes everything to work together for the good of those who love God and are called according to his purpose for them (Romans 8:28).

EPILOGUE

1. "I know the plans I have for you," says the LORD. "They are plans for good and not for disaster, to give you a future and a hope. In those days when you pray, I will listen. If you look for me wholeheartedly, you will find me" (Jeremiah 29:11-13).

Those who search will surely find me (Proverbs 8:17).

I tell you, keep on asking, and you will receive what you ask for. Keep on seeking, and you will find. Keep on knocking, and the door will be opened to you. For everyone who asks, receives. Everyone who seeks, finds. And to everyone who knocks, the door will be opened (Luke 11:9-10).

A Final Word

PRAYER IS FOR THE PATIENT, not the physician. Granted, the physician and staff may also be blessed, but prayer is for the patient.

In prayer as in surgery, where there is opportunity to do great good, there is also the potential to do harm. I don't ask to pray with everyone, because prayer with those who don't want it is neither helpful nor kind. There is no one prayer "prescription" that I advocate, except perhaps that of being open to situations in which prayer would be received as a blessing. Pushing one's personal faith on another is not recommended in any setting.

On the other hand, it seems to me that offering medical or spiritual information and considering the patient's response is caring, whereas withholding information that might help is actually uncaring. Thus I believe that prayer is one of the highest forms of kindness that I can show a person.

Some people feel uncomfortable by the mention of God in their presence. In particular, those who have been hurt by religious institutions are often especially vulnerable if those in positions of authority speak of God. Whenever offense is given, whether in medical practice or elsewhere, humility helps. This is true in all areas of life; when people sense that we genuinely care, they are more open. Let us remember that we are all on a journey, that none of us have arrived.

Whatever our profession or station in life, I believe that we all desire to make a difference in the world. In caring for the whole person in my surgical practice, I have encountered life-changing responses that go far beyond the procedures I perform. As with anything of value, though, there is a cost involved. For example, time is a limited resource; each of us is given the same daily amount. In my practice, my schedule needed to change to allow time for those in need. Through this book I hope to inspire you to approach the relationships in your own spheres of influence, whatever they are, with greater love and authenticity.

David attended medical school at Emory University School of Medicine in Atlanta, Georgia. He completed his residency in neurosurgery at Barrow Neurological Institute in Phoenix, Arizona, and did a fellowship in Endovascular Neurosurgery at the University of Vienna, in Austria. In 2007 he took a year-long sabbatical that took him to prisons and orphanages in Bolivia, Peru, and Ecuador. In recent years, David has reduced his office and operative schedule, using his off-hours to speak with his patients about forgiveness and other aids to healing. He currently practices neurosurgery in San Diego, California.